Adult aphasia

Harvey Halpern

Bobbs-Merrill Educational Publishing
Indianapolis

The Bobbs-Merrill studies in communicative disorders

Series editor
HARVEY HALPERN

Consultant of speech-communication
RUSSEL R. WINDES

The Bobbs-Merrill Company, Inc.
4300 West 62nd Street
Indianapolis, Indiana 46268

First Edition
Sixth Printing—1978
Library of Congress Catalog Card Number: 72–189018
ISBN 0–672–61280–1 (pbk)

Adult aphasia

The general purpose of this paper is to present a survey of the research in the field of aphasia. Since the literature in this field has become so extensive and varied, this review attempts to put together that body of research that seems most pertinent. This survey is geared for students, clinicians, and research workers in the field of speech pathology and is also meant to be used as a guide for source material.

Definition of aphasia

Aphasia can be defined as a multi-modality language disturbance due to brain injury. It is a linguistic deficit that causes the individual to have difficulty in the comprehension and/or formulation of language symbols. Aphasia is not generalized intellectual impairment, apraxia of speech, confused language, or dysarthria, although components of any combination of those disorders may accompany aphasic disturbance. A discussion of the differential diagnosis involved in identifying the above named disorders will be treated elsewhere in this paper.

Although there is much confusion over the terminology and nomenclature in aphasia, a few definitions seem warranted to start any discussion of aphasic disturbance. Difficulty in the comprehension of spoken language symbols is generally known as auditory aphasia. Here the individual might have greater difficulty in understanding 1.) abstract words as opposed to concrete; 2.) longer words than short; 3.) infrequently used words as compared with frequent; 4.) certain parts of speech; 5.) words that sound alike; 6.) closely associated words; and 7.) complex sentences. There can be a reduced auditory retention span and a general slowness of comprehension. Alexia is the term used when an individual has an impairment in the comprehension of written symbols (reading). Many of the same disturbances that apply to the auditory aphasic can be observed in alexia except that here the difficulty is in comprehension through the visual modality.

Difficulty in the formulation of spoken language symbols can be called oral expressive aphasia. This problem is probably influenced by the factors cited under auditory aphasia and manifests itself as a reduced vocabulary, telegraphese, jargon, agrammatisms, reduced fluency, excessive fluency, circumlocutions, neologisms, paraphasia, phonemic changes, and word finding difficulties.

An impairment in the formulation of written language symbols is called agraphia, and many of the problems and influencing factors cited in the other categories would apply here. Acalculia is a disturbance in handling numerical symbols either through comprehension in listening and/or reading, or formulation in speaking and/or writing.

Factors that influence and relate to aphasic responses will be discussed more fully in other portions of this paper.

Classification of aphasia

A number of classification systems are presented to indicate the various approaches to the categorization of aphasic disturbance.

Weisenberg and McBride (1935, p. 147) gave us one of the earliest and also one of the best known systems of aphasia classification. Their categories are as follows:

1. Predominantly Receptive: The greatest amount of disturbance is in the individual's ability to comprehend spoken or written symbols.

2. Predominantly Expressive: The greatest amount of disturbance is in the individual's ability to express ideas in speech or in writing.
3. Amnesic: The chief difficulty is in the evocation of appropriate words, as names for objects, conditions, relationships, qualities, and so on.
4. Expressive-Receptive: Both receptive and expressive language functions are extremely disturbed.

This classification system is quite popular (Osgood and Miron 1963, p. 8) and was probably made more popular because of Eisenson's adoption of the system in his widely used test called Examining for Aphasia (1954).

A more recent approach to a categorization of aphasia is the Schuell et al. (1964, chap. 9) classification system. They described 5 major categories and 2 minor syndromes. The 5 major categories are as follows:

1. Simple aphasia, defined as reduction of available language in all modalities, in the absence of specific perceptual, sensori-motor, or dysarthric components.
2. Aphasia complicated by central involvement of visual processes.
3. Aphasia with severe reduction of language in all modalities complicated by sensorimotor involvement.
4. Aphasia with some residual language preserved, and scattered findings that usually include both visual involvement and dysarthria.
5. An irreversible aphasic syndrome characterized by almost complete loss of functional language skills.

The 2 minor syndromes are described as:

a) Aphasia with partial auditory imperception, and some residual language retained or recovered early.
b) Mild aphasia with persisting dysarthria.

Schuell et al. (1964, p. 113) and Jenkins and Schuell (1964) feel that aphasia is a general language defect that crosses all language modalities and may or may not be complicated by other sequelae of brain damage. This language deficit is characterized primarily by a reduction of available vocabulary and impaired verbal retention span which is not modality specific but rather cuts across all modalities. The language deficit may or may not be complicated by additional impairment of auditory, visual, and sensorimotor processes.

Opposed to Schuell's point of view that aphasia is a general language defect that crosses all language modalities are Wepman et al. (1960), and Jones and Wepman (1961), who feel that aphasic (symbolic) disturbances are due to modality-bound input and output disturbances. They state that the agnosias and apraxias are nonsymbolic, transmissive disturbances that can, however, affect symbolization by reducing input and output capacities. From the concept that several dimensions underlie aphasic performance, Wepman and Jones (1961) have evolved a classification system of 5 categories of aphasia which are presented as follows:

1. Syntactic: where the syntax or grammar is disturbed.
2. Semantic: where the substantive language is disturbed (word-finding difficulties).
3. Pragmatic: where there is a lack of meaningful speech (no context can be found).
4. Jargon: where speech is unintelligible.
5. Global: where little or no speech is available.

Wepman and Jones (*Disorders of communication,* 1964) go on to parallel the 5 categories of aphasia with the 5 stages of language development in children. The comparison follows in this manner: speechlessness of child—global aphasia; babbling, cooing of child—jargon aphasia; fortuitous speech of child—pragmatic aphasia; substantive symbol acquisition of child—semantic aphasia; grammatical acquisition of child—syntactic aphasia. The authors conclude that recovery from aphasia should follow these stages.

Some classification systems include the site of lesion as part of their description of aphasia. The Speech Pathology Section, Aphasia Research Unit, V.A. Hospital in Boston classifies aphasics by syndromes, using classical terminology in describing the type of aphasia. The types of aphasia are Broca's, Wernicke's, Conduction, Isolation, and Anomic.

In Broca's Aphasia, the site of lesion is posterior inferior frontal, spontaneous speech is nonfluent, comprehension is intact, repetition is limited, and naming is limited.

In Wernicke's Aphasia, the site of lesion is posterior superior temporal, spontaneous speech is fluent, comprehension is impaired, repetition is impaired, and naming is impaired.

In Conduction Aphasia, the site of lesion is the arcuate fasciculus, spontaneous speech is fluent, comprehension is intact, repetition is impaired, and naming is impaired.

In Isolation Syndrome, the site of lesion is the association cortex, spontaneous speech is fluent and echolalic, comprehension is impaired, repetition is intact, and naming is impaired.

In Anomic Aphasia, the site of lesion is the angular gyrus, spontaneous speech is fluent, comprehension is intact, repetition is intact, and naming is impaired.

In another approach based on a localizationist point of view Luria (*Disorders of language,* 1964; 1970) outlines 6 categories of aphasia as follows:

1. Sensory Aphasia: This includes the symptoms of disturbance of the understanding of speech, defects in the repetition of words and the naming of objects, impairment in writing, and several distinctive defects of the patient's spontaneous speech. Locus of lesion is in the left posterior one-third of upper temporal convolution.
2. Acoustic-Amnestic Aphasia: These patients may correctly repeat phonemes similar in sound, and they lose their clear differentiation only when the amount of information impinging upon them is increased. Locus of lesion is in the left temporal area.
3. Afferent Motor Aphasia: In more severe cases of such disorders, the patient cannot find a single combination of movements needed for the pronunciation of the corresponding sound. This disturbance of the articulem constitutes a primary defect, which develops during impairment of a given area of the brain. Secondary defect (a form of efferent or kinesthetic motor aphasia) exists when the patient is not able to pronounce sounds or words using a kinesthetic foundation but may successfully compensate for this defect by using visual afferentation as a guide. Restorative work in these patients therefore uses the reconstruction of articulation on the basis of visual analysis. Locus of lesion is in the postcentral area.
4. Efferent Motor Aphasia: The patient has significant difficulty in transition from the pronunciation of separate sounds to a whole phrase, or even more to linked expression. In late stages, telegraphese may appear. Locus of lesion is Broca's Area (third frontal convolution).
5. Semantic Aphasia: Patient confuses meaning and misunderstands what you say. Locus of lesion is in the parieto-temporo-occipital areas.
6. Dynamic Aphasia: These people cannot propositionalize or have independent expression. No spontaneity of speech. Locus of lesion is in the third frontal convolution.

Jakobson (Jakobson and Halle 1956, pp. 63–75) views the classification of aphasia as a "similarity" and "contiguity" dichotomy. Patients with a similarity disorder show particular disturbances in word finding, in labeling, in initiating utterances with nominal terms, in categorizing tasks, and any task that requires spontaneous selection or substitution of lexical (semantic) items. They also display the characteristic semantic paraphasia, and, in extreme cases, may be reduced to a form of jargon in which the structure of their language is preserved but the substance is meaningless.

Patients with a contiguity disorder experience severe difficulty with combining words into more complex construction, in transforming sentences grammatically, and in rhythmic and sequential performances generally. The "little words" and grammatical tags are most susceptible to this type of disorder, the patient in the extreme cases being reduced to "telegraphese."

It is interesting to note that Jakobson (*Disorders of language*, 1964, pp. 21–46) sees an interrelationship between his dichotomy of aphasic disturbance based on linguistics and Luria's classification system based on localization theory. Jakobson likens efferent, dynamic and afferent types with contiguity disorders and the three other types in Luria's nomenclature, sensory, semantic, and acoustic-amnestic with similarity disorders.

Several approaches to classification have been presented based on the number of words that aphasic patients say. Howes (*Disorders of language*, 1964) found a range of 12 to 220 words per minute in aphasic patients, compared to a range of 100 to 175 words per minute in normal controls, and this confirmed that many aphasic patients have a distinctly sparse output of words whereas others have many words. He found two types of aphasia related to rate of output. Type A has a proportional decrease in output according to severity of the patient and is associated with anterior lesions. Type B has an increase in output of words in proportion to the clinical severity and is associated with posterior lesions.

Goodglass et al. (1964) used phrase length as the criterion measure and found that in over 90% of the cases under study, the short phrase-length group were classified clinically as Broca's aphasia, whereas the long phrase group were considered either Wernicke's or anomic types of aphasia. Benson (1967) studied 100 aphasic subjects and using a different criterion measure found that 64% of them readily fell into one of two groups. Using the radio isotope brain scan, he found that the cluster with the anterior lesion had speech characterized by low verbal output, dysprosody, dysarthria, considerable effort, and predominant use of substantive words. The posterior group were normal or near normal in all these features but often had paraphasia, press of speech, and a distinct lack of substantive words. It was felt that an anterior or posterior localization could be reliably diagnosed in many cases of aphasia based solely on the characteristics of verbal output.

Goodglass et al. (1970) investigated 52 aphasics and found that diagnostic subgroups (Wernicke's, Broca's, Conduction, anomic, and global aphasia) could be distinguished on the basis of some forms of auditory comprehension. Similarly, Goodglass and Hunter (1970) studied the speech and writing of one Wernicke's and one Broca's aphasic subject and found that they showed the same contrasting features in both medias of expression.

Bay (1966) complains about current classification systems, claiming that they are biased and inconsistent and lead to great misunderstanding of the literature. The classification system used by Bay and his colleagues has its theoretical background in the idea that aphasia should be limited to troubles that primarily and immediately concern language as a specific human function. Doing this requires the addition of categories which hold nonlinguistic status. Dysarthria, hearing loss, euphoria are examples of nonlinguistic symptoms and should be differentiated from aphasia.

Keenan (1968) feels that a receptive-expressive dichotomy is unjustified because it implies that either receptive or expressive could predominate. The author feels that all aphasic patients have more severe expressive difficulties than receptive ones and cites the work done on the Minnesota Test For Differential Diagnosis of Aphasia and the Language Modalities Test for Aphasia where expressive scores were much lower than receptive scores. In a number of articles Critchley (1967; 1970) traces the nomenclature, derivation of terms, and classifications used in aphasia.

It is apparent from the classification systems reviewed that no clear pattern emerges but rather a mass of overlapping and conflicting views. Criticism of the expressions "expressive" and "receptive" to describe aphasic language behavior has ranged from the comment that this dichotomy is too vague and noncommittal to the statement that these two designations are not comparable to each other. As stated earlier, Schuell's ideas have been attacked for claiming that aphasia is a general language defect that crosses all language modalities.

Wepman and Jones have been criticized for their views that state that aphasic disturbances are due to modality-bound input and output disturbances. The parallel of their 5 categories of aphasia with the 5 stages of language development in children appears to need further proof.

Classification systems that use classical terminology seem to fall into "pure" types and nomenclature problems. For example, it's not clear whether apraxia of speech is only seen as part of "Broca's aphasia" or whether apraxia of speech is the condition called "Motor aphasia."

While Jakobson's hypothesis of a "continguity" and "similarity" dichotomy of aphasic language behavior is quite exciting, further substantiating evidence of this theory is needed. Finally, systems based on the number of words aphasic subjects say seem to get stalled with the "type B" patient where the wide discrepancy of language behavior between a mild and severe patient is not fully explained.

One way to work out of this morass of overlapping and conflicting views is to first make sure that you're looking at an aphasic patient. Too often what is assumed to be aphasia could be the speech and language behavior of other brain-injury syndromes. Earlier in this paper it was stated that aphasia is not a generalized intellectual impairment, apraxia of speech, confused language, or dysarthria, although components of any combination of those disorders may accompany aphasic disturbance. A look at those other speech and language disorders will reveal why a distinction must be made in any scheme for identifying aphasic language disturbance.

A generalized intellectual impairment implies a general lowering of intellectual functions. Performance on language tasks and nonmental tasks are about the same and lowered. The patient usually exhibits an "across the board" depression of mental faculties, personality changes, emotional lability, dull and bland behavior, and memory loss (Darley 1964, p. 39; Mayo Clinic 1964, pp. 238–239; Halpern et al. 1969). This disorder can resemble a mild aphasia.

Apraxia of speech is an articulation disorder that results from impairment due to brain damage, of the capacity to order the positioning of speech musculature and the sequencing of muscle movements for volitional production of phonemes and sequences of phonemes; but it is not accompanied by significant weakness, slowness, or incoordination of these same muscles in reflex and automatic acts (Darley 1964, p. 36; Johns and Darley 1970). This disorder can resemble a good deal of the oral expressive language behavior of the aphasic patient. For example, the phonemic groping of the apraxic patient can resemble the word-finding difficulty of the aphasic patient.

Confused language is part of a condition where the patient's responsiveness to his environment is impaired to a mild degree. Psychological responses are slower, restricted in scope, and less adaptive. The behavior indicates that the patient is less able to recognize and understand the environment than in the normal state. Clearness of thinking and accuracy of remembering are impaired. The patient usually manifests a disorientation of time and place, confabulations, an inability to follow directions, and is unaware of the inappropriateness of his responses (Darley 1964, pp. 38–39; Mayo Clinic 1964, p. 234; Halpern et al. 1969). The bizarre, irrelevant responses typical of this disorder can easily resemble the responses of the aphasic patient who has a marked difficulty in comprehending spoken language. This type of aphasic patient will emit jargon or paraphasic responses much like that in the language of confusion.

Dysarthria is a collective name for a group of speech disorders resulting from disturbance in muscular control over the speech mechanism due to damage of the central or peripheral nervous system. It designates problems in oral communication due to slowness, weakness, or incoordination of the speech musculature (Darley et al. 1969a,b). Dysarthria can resemble certain manifestations of oral expressive aphasia.

Once we have identified and recognized these related syndromes, could we not view aphasia as a unified disorder instead of resorting to all sorts of overlapping divisions within the disorder? This unified approach, which emphasizes that aphasic disturbances affects all the language modalities, has been elaborated on by Schuell et al. (1964, p. 113) and brought into focus by a recent study by Smith (1971). He found that standardized language tests of 78 stroke patients with chronic aphasia revealed patterns of associated defects in speech, auditory comprehension, reading, and writing that did not coincide with the traditional dichotomy of Broca's "motor" vs Wernicke's "sensory" (or other classical, anatomically based classifications of) aphasia as originally described. Although the nature and degree of impairment in the four language components may vary in chronic aphasia, all four language components are generally impaired.

In this manner, one would first diagnose the speech and language behavior as being aphasia, or aphasia with apraxia of speech, or aphasia with confused language, etc. After such a diagnosis, a description of the speech and language problems in the various modalities would be given. "Pure" types or dichotomous breakdowns would not be necessary since evidence is mounting that aphasic language disturbance cuts across all modalities in different patterns.

Maybe we ought to view the "pure" types as those who have just aphasia without any accompanying speech and language disturbance, and the "mixed" types as those who have aphasia with an additional speech and language syndrome.

Disorders related to aphasia

Quite often aphasia is accompanied by disturbances that are nonlinguistic in nature. These disturbances are the apraxias, the agnosias, and the dysarthrias, and not only can they confound and resemble aphasia but they must be differentiated from aphasia for diagnostic and therapeutic purposes.

Apraxia Apraxia is defined by Nielsen (1946, p. 59) as a disturbance in which a patient without dementia, incoordination, or paralysis is nevertheless, because of a motor incapacity, unable to apply his powers to voluntary purposes. Apraxia is usually caused by a brain lesion and as Wepman et al. (1960) state, it is a nonsymbolic transmissive type of disorder.

In the early 1900s, Liepmann (Weisenberg and McBride 1935, pp. 104–105) stated that types of apraxia showing a predominance of "motor" symptoms are related to more anterior lesions while "ideational" forms are said to be caused by lesions more posterior in the brain. He delineated a limb-kinetic, an ideo-kinetic, and an ideational apraxia. Limb-kinetic apraxia exists when the patient appreciates the nature of the movement but lacks the skill and is slow and awkward in the performance of the activity. Liepmann postulated a loss of kinesthetic engrams as a possible cause. With ideo-kinetic apraxia the patient has difficulty in determining what the nature of a simple movement shall be. Many times the patient has forgotten how to use particular tools for movements, and as a result they may take place haphazardly. There seems to be a break between the kinesthetic process and ideation. With ideational apraxia the patient has a faulty conception of the movement as a whole with temporal and spatial relationships confused.

In 1922 Kleist (Weisenberg and McBride, p. 105) described constructional apraxia as a break in visuo-kinesthetic connections. The patient experiences difficulty in laying out sticks to copy a given design, in building with blocks, in drawing, in writing, and sometimes in placing block letters to form words. He may show that he has a concept of the object he is to draw, which fails only in spatial orientation or in spatial relationship of the parts.

Ettlinger (1969) suggests in a theoretical paper that the neurological condition normally termed apraxia consists of two separate components. First, a disorder in the execution of verbal commands. This disorder can be termed "language dependent" and is thought to be necessarily associated with pathology of the major hemisphere. Second, a disorder of the ability to copy movements demonstrated by the examiner and associated sometimes with the defective use of objects. This disorder should be distinguished from apraxia proper and is thought to be a consequence of bilateral pathology.

Benson and Barton (1970) tested 24 subjects with positive radio-active brain scans in one of 4 quadrants of the brain (right anterior, right posterior, left anterior, left posterior) and 16 patients with no evidence of focal brain damage on a battery of 6 tests to assess constructional ability. There is evidence that lesions in the right hemisphere produce more consistent disturbances in visuo-spatial tasks than do similar lesions in the left hemisphere, and that there is a greater consistency of performance with posterior lesions (in either hemisphere) than with anteriorly located lesions. This article also presents a comprehensive historical review of research done in constructional apraxia.

Although the work done by Liepmann and Kleist centered mainly on apraxia of the limbs, they did recognize that an apraxia of speech musculature could produce certain disorders of articulation.

Apraxia of speech Recently, Darley (1969) scrutinized case reports beginning with Broca in 1861 through studies done by Johns and Darley (1970) and Shankweiler et al. (1968) and found several characteristic behavioral strands that preserve the identity and continuity of a disorder which he called apraxia of speech. Darley describes the characteristics of apraxia of speech as follows:

1. Phonemic errors are prominent with omissions, substitutions, distortions, additions, and repetitions of phonemes.
2. Some errors appear to be perseverative, others anticipatory.
3. Errors are seemingly off-target approximations of the desired production made in an effortful groping for the correct position or sequence of positions.
4. Errors are highly inconsistent, unlike those of dysarthria.
5. Errors vary with the complexity of the articulatory adjustment.
6. Errors increase as words increase in length.
7. There is a discrepancy between the articulatory accuracy displayed in

automatic-reactive speech performance and the inaccuracy displayed in volitional-purposive performances.

8. Imitative responses are particularly poor.
9. The speaker is usually aware of his errors but is typically unable to anticipate or correct them.
10. Monitoring of speech in anticipation of errors leads to prosodic disturbances such as slowed rate, even stress, even spacing.
11. Oral apraxia is often, but not always, observed in association with apraxia of speech.

Darley feels that these distinctive characteristics warrant the adoption of a terminology that differentiates this disorder clearly from problems due to muscular weakness or incoordination (dysarthria) and from problems due to inefficient processing of linguistic units (aphasia). A separate term, apraxia of speech, best denotes the dynamics of the problem and obviates the necessity for an intervening step of redescription often resorted to when terms like "cortical dysarthria" or "motor aphasia" are used.

The necessity to use a separate term, apraxia of speech, instead of terms that need redescription seems quite obvious when one looks at the literature. Some of the following studies use terms such as articulatory dyspraxia, cortical dysarthria, phonemic-articulatory disorders, and verbal apraxia, which in all probability actually describe the condition called apraxia of speech.

Critchley (1952) stated that many asphasic patients show disorders of articulate speech that are both varied and variable in their character. Dysarthria and dysphasia, though often occurring in combination, are actually separate phenomena. Articulatory dyspraxia is also an independent entity, although it may coexist with an aphasia and contribute to defects of articulation. Bay (1964) reported on a study of 80 unselected aphasic patients and found a well defined and frequent group of speech disorders marked by a distinct apraxia of the articulatory muscles and impaired tongue movements in the glossogram test. Bay says he is describing what other people have referred to as motor aphasia, but what he calls "cortical dysarthria." His main point is that it is a motor disorder independent of language, and we must distinguish this motor disorder from the linguistic disorders called aphasia.

DeRenzi et al. (1966) tested 105 aphasic patients, and they found a high correlation between the severity of oral apraxia and the severity of phonemic-articulatory disorder; oral apraxia and Broca's aphasia were a common combination; oral apraxia was present in about one-third of conduction aphasics and usually absent in Wernicke's aphasia; oral apraxia was not considered to be a part of a general praxic disturbance.

Canter (1969), in a position paper, looks at verbal apraxia as a primary and secondary dichotomy. Primary verbal apraxia is characterized by damage to the region of Broca's area, reduced phonemic repetoires, and articulation errors with sound substitutions and distortions that can be described in terms of closeness to the place and manner of articulation of the intended sound. Secondary verbal apraxia is characterized by damage to sensory association areas or transcortical tracts, and articulatory errors tend to be based on incorrect phoneme selection and on errors in sequencing phonemes and syllables. The sound selection errors are often not as reasonable as those observed in primary verbal apraxia; that is, there may be little phonetic similarity between the sound intended and the sound actually produced.

Johns and Darley (1970) studied 10 apraxic of speech and 10 dysarthric subjects and found that these patients typically display marked discrepancy between good perception of stimuli and poor oral production of the same stimuli. Specific phonemes do not differentiate dysarthric and apraxic patients but types of errors and their consistency do: dysarthric patients showed predominantly distortions and unrelated substitutions, whereas apraxic patients showed predominantly unrelated substitutions, repetitions, and additions. The mode of stimulus presentation affects performance: auditory-visual is better than auditory or visual alone. Few errors are simplification, suggesting inappropriateness of the term "phonetic disintegration."

In a follow-up study that utilized the same 10 patients with apraxia of speech as Johns and Darley (1970), Aten et al. (1971) found that apraxia of speech patients made significantly more auditory perceptual errors as a group than normal subjects but varied considerably in their level of performance. The achievement of some patients was within the range established by the control subjects; that of others was unequivocally inferior. The major deficit in the apraxic group appeared to be impairment of ability to retain the second and third syllable consonant elements in three-word sequences.

Although the research reviewed is plagued by nomenclature problems, it is obvious that a condition known as apraxia of speech exists. This condition can exist as a separate entity without aphasia or it can coexist with aphasia. This author firmly believes in its existence, and a further elaboration of this condition can be found in the sections dealing with "phonemic regression" and "differential diagnosis."

Agnosia Agnosia, a disturbance of recognition or identification of sensory stimuli, can accompany aphasia, and has been described by Wepman et al. (1960) as a nonsymbolic transmissive type of disorder. Brain (1961, chapter 14) has outlined the following common forms of agnosia.

Auditory agnosia occurs when a patient with unimpaired hearing fails to recognize or identify the sounds which he hears. He may have difficulty recognizing the difference between familiar noises such as the crumpling of paper, the jingling of money, bells, sirens, tires screeching, etc. Auditory agnosia can also involve the identification of spoken speech and thus lead to pure-word deafness, and may be accompanied by difficulty in recognizing musical sounds or sensory amusia.

Visual agnosia is present when the patient has difficulty in recognizing objects he sees when this can not be attributed either to defects of visual acuity or to generalized intellectual impairment. A number of forms of visual agnosia have been delineated: 1.) visual agnosia for objects or visual object-agnosia; 2.) simultanagnosia, or the failure to appreciate the meaning of a picture though its individual elements are correctly identified; 3.) visual agnosia for colors; 4.) visual agnosia for space. If the patient has difficulty in identifying printed letters or words, a condition known as pure word-blindness occurs.

Tactile agnosia refers to a disturbance in the ability to recognize and identify objects by means of touch when both the superficial and deep sensibility of the part of the body to be tested are normal. Coins, combs, scissors, and other common objects are used for identifying purposes.

A rather odd combination of agnosic and aphasic difficulties can be found in Gerstmann's Syndrome (Brain 1961, p. 168). It is described as the patient having finger agnosia, a right-left disorientation, agraphia, and acalculia. However, the authenticity and isolation of this syndrome has been questioned by Benton (1959), Critchley (1966), and Poeck and Orgass (1966).

Further information concerning the various subtypes, locus of lesion, and additional nomenclature involving agnosia can be found in Nielsen (1946) and Brain (1961). Testing procedures for the agnosias will be found in the Diagnosis section of this paper.

Dysarthria Many times a condition known as dysarthria will accompany the aphasic disorder. As described earlier, Darley et al. (1969a,b) state that dysarthria is a collective name for a group of speech disorders resulting from disturbances in muscular control over the speech mechanism due to damage of the central or peripheral nervous system. It designates problems in oral communication due to slowness, weakness, or incoordination of the speech musculature. It differentiates such problems from disorders of higher centers related to the faulty programming of movements and sequences of movements (apraxia of speech) and to the inefficient processing of linguistic units (aphasia).

In a further explanation of the problem, Darley et al. (1969a,b) studied 212 patients, and five types of dysarthria were delineated: flaccid dysarthria (in bulbar palsy), spastic dysarthria (in pseudo-bulbar palsy), ataxic dysarthria (in cerebellar disorders), hypokinetic dysarthria (in parkinsonism), and hyperkinetic dysarthria (in dystonia and chorea). In addition, a mixed dysarthria combining the elements of flaccid and spastic dysarthrias has been identified in amyotrophic lateral sclerosis.

Differential factors involved in dysarthria and other speech and language syndromes are further discussed in the section called differential diagnosis.

Historical review

An analysis of the literature on aphasia from Hippocratic writings to 1800 by Benton and Joynt (1960) reveals that a substantial amount of knowledge about many clinical forms of aphasia was already in existence at the time of Hippocrates. A number of reviews by Nielsen (1946, chap. 1), Baker (1954), Penfield and Roberts (1959, chap. 4), Brain (1961, chap. 4), Schuell et al. (1964, chaps. 1, 2, 3), and Critchley (1970, chaps. 5, 6, 7, 8, 9) trace the history and thought of aphasia from 1800 to the present. It is recounted here in condensed form:

Gall, in 1810, was the first man to relate speech to a particular area of the brain and one of the early localizationists. In his description of two cases, Gall postulated an organ for words and language in the anterior portions of the brain. Spurzheim was a student of Gall's from 1810 to 1819 and agreed with him. He stated that there was one area for learning artificial signs and that this area was in the anterior portion of the brain. Bell, in 1811, demonstrated the differentiation of sensory and motor nerves and indicated that the brain was localized for certain functions and had autonomous centers. Bouillaud, in 1825, studied 850 cases and found lesions in the frontal lobes of 116 patients who were speech defective. He postulated a "faculty of speech" and felt that if localization were not true, hemiparesis could not occur.

Opposed to this early localization point of view was Flourens, who stated in 1824 that all parts of the brain were equipotential and that specific areas for specific purposes did not exist. If an area was damaged because of disease or injury, any other area of the brain could take over that function.

Dax, in 1836, collected more than 30 cases showing that loss of speech and paresis of the right side were due to damage in the left hemisphere. Joynt and Benton (1964) note that a full English translation of the 1836 memoir indicates that Dax reported the association between aphasic disorders and lesions of the left hemisphere prior to Broca. However, those authors conclude that Dax was unwilling to take public responsibility and thus recorded it in the form of an essentially private communication, which was published in 1865, after Dax's death, by his physician son, Gustav.

In 1861, Broca (Penfield and Roberts, 1959, chap. 4), on the basis of two cases, said that the "motor speech area" was located in the third frontal convolution. Critics of Broca's findings argue that there was no proof that the lesion in the third frontal was the oldest, examination of the patient was inadequate according to present day standards, and that neither brain was sectioned so that any anatomic conclusion is unjustifiable. Broca postulated that there were four fundamentals involved in the production of speech. 1.) Ideas; their loss would lead to alogia (mental retardation?). 2.) Connection between ideas and words; a disruption of this connection would give verbal amnesia (Aphasia?). 3.) Combination of movements of the articulators with suitable words; a disturbance of this would cause aphemia or loss of speech (Apraxia of Speech?). 4.) Use of organs of articulation; its loss would lead to mechanical alalia (Dysarthria?). At the centenary of Broca's work, Joynt (1961) wrote a comprehensive review of Broca's contributions.

Trousseau, in 1861, argued with Broca's use of the term aphemia (loss of speech) and said that it really meant infamy. Trousseau gave us the term aphasia (loss of speech) and said it was caused by damage in the third frontal convolution, Island of Reil, and the corpus striatum. Ogle, in 1867, called Broca's Syndrome "ataxic aphasia" and said that every individual must have a memory of muscular movements plus a memory for words. He gave us the term "agraphia," which meant a disturbance in writing.

In 1869, Bastian was one of the first in a school of thought to be known later as "strict localizationists." He was the first to describe "word deafness and word blindness," and he believed that one thought in words and that there were four different specific centers in the brain with fibre connections. These centers were the auditory, visual, glosso-kinesthetic (motor speech), and cheiro-kinesthetic (motor writing). Bastian felt that there were no true motor areas in the cortex but that they existed instead in the medulla and the spinal cord. He thought the cortex was sensory in function and that speech functions were psychical products of specific anatomical cerebral areas, with specific cerebral areas for specific images.

In 1874, Wernicke, a young genius, studied 3 cases and designated the rear of the first temporal convolution as the auditory interpretation area. He stated that damage to this area would result in the patient's inability to interpret auditorily and would also interfere with reading and writing. He felt that people learn these two functions through the auditory modality. Wernicke labeled this impairment sensory aphasia. He further stated that anterior portions of the brain were devoted to motor functions and posterior portions to sensory functions. Wernicke accepted Broca's area but suggested that there were fibres connecting Broca's area and the first temporal convolution. If injured, they would produce conduction aphasia, which is characterized by a marked paraphasia. Geschwind (1967b) has written a comprehensive review of Wernicke's contribution to the study of aphasia.

In 1877, Kussmaul, a localizationist, said that the visual speech or reading center was located in the angular gyrus. He gave us a classification of aphasia which consisted of: a) ataxic aphasia, b) amnesic aphasia, c) dumbness for words, d) paraphasia, e) agrammatism and akataphasia. Broadbent, in 1878, was one of the same school of "localizationists," and he introduced the concept of "anomia." He described visual, auditory, tactile, and speech centers, as well as naming and propositionizing (intellectual) centers. In 1885, Lichtheim, a localizationist, described visual, auditory, motor, and writing plus ideational centers. He also thought of psychical images related to cerebral centers. In 1887, Charcot, another localizationist, said that a word consisted of 4 distinct memories of images and that they were auditory, visual, motor articulatory, and graphic. He said that these areas were autonomous of each other but that in various individuals different centers predominated in the functioning of internal speech. Charcot spoke convincingly of visual and auditory mindedness and of psychical images related to specific cerebral areas.

Strongly opposed to the rather prevalent localizationist theories of the time was an independent Englishman named Hughlings Jackson. Jackson (Head 1926, vol. 1) started publishing his thoughts in 1864 and asserted that the patient does not lose the faculty of speech but rather loses the power to use words in propositions. He favored the dynamic concept of speech activities and said that there were three different psychological levels of language. 1.) Utterances that were not speech. 2.) Utterances that were inferior speech (oaths, exclamations, etc.). 3.) True speech or utterances that expressed relationships. Jackson saw aphasia on the third or last level and said that destructive lesions never cause positive effects but induce a negative condition that permits positive symptoms to appear. The loss of speech is really the loss of power to propositionalize aloud. Negative symptoms consist mainly of an inability to speak, write, read, and pantomime. Positive symptoms are the ability to understand what is said or read to one and the ability to use emotional language.

Jackson postulated that the left hemisphere is used for articulatory movements and imitation of speech and that the right hemisphere is used for the reception of speech, images, or symbols and is responsible for automatic speech, jargon, etc. (positive symptoms). He stressed that language is in large part psychological and not purely physiological, and in light of this he urged not only the study of the anatomy of the cerebrum at autopsy but also that of the live patient. Riese (1965) offers a further elaboration of Jackson's view on aphasia.

Marie, in 1906, denied that a damaged third frontal lobe caused aphasia but said that damage to the lenticular nucleus (essential to motor speech), along with damage to the third frontal lobe, caused anarthria. He stated that true aphasia was damage to Wernicke's area and denied the concept of auditory and visual image centers because of the great variability in aphasic symptoms. Marie stated that aphasic symptoms were due to a decrease in general intelligence and that anarthria, which was the old subcortical motor aphasia, could exist in isolation. He said Broca's Aphasia was really his anarthria plus Wernicke's Aphasia, and he claimed that all aphasic patients have some defect in comprehension. Marie further stated that the only true aphasia was Wernicke's Aphasia, which produced poor comprehension, paraphasia, jargon, and reading and writing difficulties. Cole (1968) presents some additional insight and concepts concerning Marie's work.

Henschen, a strict localizationist in the early 1920s, gathered and summarized about 1500 cases. He thought it was possible to localize every type of abstract thought anatomically. He called this concept physiological functioning and stated that a center was considered as a cerebral area, which produced certain pathological anomalies of behavior if damaged or destroyed. A center was not an independent entity responsible for a specific function, but damage to a center resulted in predictable changes in the execution of certain performances. He believed that bilateral destruction would knock out a function completely; therefore, if damage is only on one side (left), a person retains some language ability and can be rehabilitated because the right hemisphere is still functioning.

Head (1926, vol. 1) was an adherent of Jackson, a nonlocalizationist, and opposed the concept of pure aphasic disturbances. He stated that aphasia is not a disorder on the motor or sensory level (pure), but rather a difficulty in using motor and sensory performances in a symbolic fashion. He describes symbolic formulation and expression as any kind of behavior in which some verbal or other symbol intervenes between the commencing and ending of an act. Aphasia and apraxia have no direct causal relationship, since apraxia is a disturbance on a strictly motor level. He noted that aphasics had difficulty not only with language but also with numbers, pictures, the alphabet, letters, coins, etc. when used symbolically.

Head strongly believed in the psychological aspects of language and aphasia and noticed that patients could do particular things at one time and not another, probably for psychological reasons. He proposed four categories of aphasia: Verbal Aphasia, Syntactical Aphasia, Nominal Aphasia, and Semantic Aphasia.

a) Verbal Aphasia can be caused by lesions affecting the lower portions of the precentral and postcentral convolutions. The patient has defective ability to form words, whether for external or internal use.

b) Syntactical Aphasia can be caused by lesions affecting the upper convolutions of the temporal lobe. The patient lacks balance and rhythm in speech. He displays telegraphese, jargon, logarrhea, etc.

c) Nominal Aphasia can be caused by lesions affecting the angular gyrus area. Here the patient has difficulty with the names of things.

d) Semantic Aphasia can be caused by lesions affecting the supramarginal gyrus. The patient confuses meaning and misunderstands what you say.

Nielsen (1946) is a present-day localizationist who has delineated 87 different types of aphasia, agnosia, and apraxia with their locus of lesion. Nielsen was strongly influenced by the work of Henschen and thus saw aphasia in a neurophysiological framework. His text *Agnosia, Apraxia, Aphasia* is a modern-day classic of the cerebral localization school. Olsen (1963) has sketched a biography of Nielsen that also contains a complete bibliography of Nielsen's work and other literature dealing with the localizationist point of view.

Lashley, in work done over the last 25 years, opposes localization and says that complex mental functions are the result of the entire cerebrum functioning and not of specific structural entities. As a result of his experiments with rats, Lashley conceived the concept of Mass Action. This concept states that retarding effects of lesions were equal in different parts of the rat's brain responsible for highly integrated units of behavior. He further explained that all parts of the brain operated equally and that there existed, within specialized areas, a principle of "equi-potentiality," i.e. subordinate parts of the specialized area could produce independently the intact function of the whole specialized area. The amount of cerebrum left intact counted more than the site of the lesion.

Kurt Goldstein (1948, chap. 1), whose work in aphasia ranged from pre-World War I through the 1960s, felt that the workings of the brain can be likened to the concept of "figure-ground" relationship. The "figure" standing for a particular area playing a major role and the rest of the brain acting as the "background." If injury occurs, this balance is upset. The symptoms due to de-differentiation (disintegration) of function may impair a person's ability to abstract, and Goldstein postulated that the abstract attitude is needed for the following:

Assuming a mental set voluntarily to begin a performance Here the patient may have trouble initiating speech but will do so if he is started off with a word or a sound.

Shifting voluntarily from one aspect to another An example would be shifting from counting numbers to recitation of the alphabet or from saying the days of the week to saying the months of the year.

Keeping in mind various aspects of a situation The aphasic patient would have difficulty with a long sentence; he would probably also lack a sense of humor because of the sudden switch in the frame of reference that characterizes a "punch line."

Grasping the essential of a given whole and its parts Examples would be knowing one room in a house or hospital but not relating it to other rooms in the house, or being unable to put a puzzle together from its parts.

Ability to see common factors in somewhat different situations This deals with placing things in categories, such as writing tools, eating tools, furniture, cars, etc. The patient would also have difficulty in pretending and make-believe situations.

Excessive ego orientation The aphasic wants all material things to touch upon himself. He will only talk about his own operation, what he did, etc.

Geschwind (1964) and Quadfasel (1968) have offered reviews of Kurt Goldstein's contributions in the field of aphasia.

Penfield (Penfield and Roberts, 1959) does not believe in pure forms of aphasia or exclusively functioning centers of control. In addition to Broca's Area and Wernicke's Area, Penfield found a third area for speech, the supplementary motor area or superior speech area (near the motor cortex for foot movement).

He said there are four areas devoted to the motor control of speech and three areas for ideational aspects. Penfield used an electrical probe on awake patients who were undergoing brain surgery. Vocalization was produced by stimulating the precentral Rolandic gyrus (near face and lip area) in both hemispheres and in the supplementary motor area (near motor foot area) in both hemispheres. Penfield found that excision of one precentral Rolandic gyrus on either side will produce temporary dysarthria. Excision of either one of the supplementary motor areas will not produce paralysis of the limbs or mouth, but if it occurs in the dominant hemisphere, it will produce temporary aphasia.

Three ideational areas were outlined by Penfield, and he found them organized for function in one hemisphere only. They consisted of the Anterior (Broca's) Area, Posterior (Wernicke's) Area, and Superior (Supplementary Speech) Area. He noted that excision of the superior area produced temporary aphasia. Excision of the anterior area caused aphasia that cleared up in some cases. Excision of the posterior area resulted in the gravest aphasia. Because excisions all around the anterior and posterior speech areas did not cause aphasia, it was assumed that these areas are connected to subcortical areas (thalamus). Penfield postulated that there are no areas for the ideational mechanism of speech on the nondominant side, but removal of the corresponding posterior speech area of the nondominant hemisphere produces apractognosia (loss of body scheme and spatial relationships about it). Total destruction of the posterior speech area in the dominant hemisphere or in the underlying posterior portion of the thalamus would produce global aphasia. In children, the opposite hemisphere will take over if the posterior area is damaged. For adults, the take-over of one area of the brain for another is still unclear.

This brief historical review was intended to show some of the thinking in aphasiology over the last 175 years. Although the work of several prominent contributors not mentioned here is noted elsewhere in this paper, some were not mentioned at all. It would be beyond the realm of this review to include all who have made contributions in the field of aphasia.

Etiology of aphasia

As was stated in the definition, aphasia is caused by brain injury. A major cause of aphasia in middle and old age is the cerebro-vascular accident. It consists of thromboses, embolisms, aneurysms, hemorrhages, and ischemias. A cerebral thrombosis is an occlusion of an artery to the brain by a clot. A cerebral embolus is a clot formed elsewhere that finally lodges in the brain. An aneurysm is a swelling or ballooning of a cranial artery. A cerebral hemorrhage is the rupture of a blood vessel with subsequent bleeding into the brain. Ischemia refers to deficient circulation in the brain. All of the cerebro-vascular accidents have one thing in common: they deprive the brain of oxygen and circulation, thus causing brain damage.

Trauma to the brain is another major cause of aphasia. Gun shot wounds, automobile accidents, and falls are most likely involved in physical trauma to the brain. Brain tumors, both malignant and nonmalignant, are associated with causing aphasia. Quite often the extirpation of a brain tumor will cause aphasia. Abscesses, infectious diseases, and degenerative diseases of the brain can also result in aphasia.

Cerebral dominance

Although it is generally accepted that a lesion on the left side of the brain in a right-handed individual will result in aphasia, some widely divergent interpretations have sprung from this concept. Taking an extreme point of view, Penfield and Roberts (1959, p. 137) stated that the left hemisphere is usually dominant for speech regardless of handedness, except for those who have had early cerebral injuries. They found no differences in the frequency of aphasia after an operation on the left side between left- and right-handed individuals. In a similar stance, Russell and Espir (1961, p. 30) indicated that speech is almost always represented in the left hemisphere, even in left-handed subjects, and that it is very rare for aphasia to follow penetrating missile wounds of the right hemisphere.

Another less extreme approach states that language representation is not always completely lateralized in one hemisphere. Jackson (Head, 1926, vol. 1) stated that the right hemisphere in right-handed persons produced nonpropositional speech, such as jargon and automatic speech, and is used for the reception of speech, while the left hemisphere is used for articulatory movements and the initiation of speech. Weisenberg and McBride (1935, p. 453) indicated that the right hemisphere is concerned with language, but to a limited degree. They worked with right brain-injured persons and found mental deterioration but not aphasia.

Milner et al. (*Disorders of language*, 1964) surveyed a number of studies which revealed that the hemisphere dominant for language is not that clear for left-handed or ambidextrous individuals. They reviewed several investigations using the Wada technique of intracarotid injection of sodium amytol, the right and left sides being injected on different days. By temporarily interfering with, in turn, the functioning of each hemisphere it is possible to compare the two cerebral hemispheres of the same patient with respect to their involvement in speech. Their review of the literature, in addition to their own study in which 123 patients were studied with the Wada technique, indicated that the cerebral organization of language is less predictable in left-handed and ambidextrous persons than in right handers.

Rossi and Rossadini (*Brain mechanisms underlying speech and language*, 1967) used intracarotid amibarbital injections and also found that hemisphere dominance for speech was rather clear for right-handed individuals but not as conclusive in left-handed and ambidextrous persons. They also felt that moods and emotions had hemispheric specialization in certain individuals, and they presented a review of the literature on this aspect. Gloning et al. (1969) presented paired data from 57 right-handed and 57 nonright-handed patients with almost identical anatomically verified cerebral lesions. Aphasic disturbances were observed in patients with both left and right hemispheric lesions. These findings support the hypothesis that most nonright-handed patients show less marked dominance for language than right-handed patients. The nonright-handed patients, do not, however, represent a uniform group, and some significant differences in language disturbance were found, depending on which hand is used for writing.

Several approaches not dealing with expressive language in cerebral lateralization have come forward. Teuber (*Brain mechanisms underlying speech and language*, 1967) has reviewed the work done on the "spatial tasks" function of the right hemisphere. Kimura (1967), after a number of her own investigations, reviews the evidence relating lateral asymmetry in auditory perception to the asymmetrical functioning of the two hemispheres of the brain. Because each ear has greater neural representation in the opposite cerebral hemisphere, the predominance of the left hemisphere for speech is reflected in superior recognition for words arriving at the right ear, while the predominance of the right hemisphere in melodic-pattern perception is reflected in superior identification of melodies arriving at the left ear.

Rubino (1970) tested non-brain-damaged left temporal and right temporal subjects and found that left temporal subjects displayed a deficit in the identification (visual) of words and that the right temporal subjects displayed a deficit in the identification of figures. Both of these experimental groups were inferior to the non-brain-damaged subjects. This study suggested that the right temporal lobe is responsible for nonverbal functioning and the left temporal for verbal functioning.

Giannitrapani (1967) traces the historical sequence of ideas that eventually led to the discovery of the medullary crossing of the pyramids, describes the difficulties surrounding the acceptance of unilateral speech representation, the subsequent hemisphere dominance notion, the current neuropathological evidence questioning such ideas, and EEG findings including EEG phase analysis data. Osgood and Miron (1963, chap. 3) present some interesting thoughts on the whole concept of cerebral dominance. A bibliography on dichotic listening has been presented by Richardson and Knights (1970).

In summation, it appears that some researchers feel that only the left hemisphere is dominant for speech regardless of handedness; some feel that the left hemisphere is dominant for speech in right-handed individuals but that dominance is not clear for those who are left-handed or ambidextrous; and some feel that the left hemisphere is dominant for speech in right-handed individuals but that most non-right-handed individuals show less marked dominance for speech in comparison with the right-handed. In addition, the studies reviewed have shown that the reception of speech is primarily located in the left hemisphere while the right hemisphere is dominant for nonverbal tasks.

Cerebral localization

Concepts of cerebral localization have been an integral part of aphasiology for almost 200 years. Some of the thinking on localization is mentioned in the "historical review" and "cerebral dominance" sections of this paper. A comprehensive treatment of the subject is presented by Hecaen and Angelergues (*Disorders of language,* 1964). They trace the history of thought on localization and also try to explain localization concepts according to vascular lesions, traumatic lesions, and stimulations and cortical excisions. In addition, they present their own material, which is based upon observation of 214 right-handed patients with lesions of the left hemisphere. All of their cases were verified either by postmortem examination or by surgery. Their anatomo-clinical observations included the patients' ability in articulation, speech fluency, verbal comprehension, naming, repetition, reading, and writing.

After carefully reviewing other studies in the area, and as a result of their own detailed study, they concluded the following concepts of localization theory. There exists

1. A central zone traditionally known as Wernicke's Zone. An impairment of it can affect all language modalities, including motor elements.
2. An anterior motor pole, which appears to be located around the lower part of the rolandic convolution in frontal and parietal areas.
3. A posterior pole affecting reading, which can itself be subdivided into two poles, one of which (lingual gyrus) is more visuo-verbal, and the other (angular gyrus), more visuo-graphic.
4. A superior pole (parietal lobe), which controls praxic activities.

In a study of 40 cerebrally involved patients, Halpern et al. (1969) found that aphasic subjects revealed a predominance of lesions posterior to the central fissure. Subjects with generalized intellectual impairment showed a predominance of diffuse lesions. Subjects who were designated as apraxic of speech patients showed a predominance of lesions anterior to the central fissure. Confused language subjects revealed a predominance of disseminated lesions.

Additional reviews, concepts and studies of localization can be found in Nielsen (1946), Goldstein (1948), Penfield and Roberts (1959), Brain (1961), Russell and Espir (1961), Sklar (1963), Osgood and Miron (1963), Luria (*Disorders of language,* 1964), Serafetinides (1966), in *Brain mechanisms underlying speech and language* (Millikan and Darley 1967), and Luria (1970).

Parameters of study in aphasia

Various studies and theoretical positions have been presented concerning the language behavior of aphasics as related to frequency of occurrence, parts of speech, abstraction level of words, word length, grammatical classes, and the concept of "phonemic regression." These parameters of language appear to influence aphasic language behavior.

Frequency of occurrence Weisenberg and McBride (1935, pp. 387–388) suggested that in treating aphasic patients, drills for word formation should at first be composed of the most frequently used words in the language. Goldstein (1948, p. 337) had also pointed out that words selected for the aphasic patient should be words that are easy to recognize visually and that are frequently used in reading.

During the past few years, attention has been given to the frequency of words in language usage as a variable in studying dysphasic speech performance. Thurston (1954) found that aphasic subjects did poorly on oral spelling tasks as the words became more difficult (less frequently used). Wepman et al. (1956) studied the speech of an anomic aphasic subject and that of a normal person and hypothesized that anomia may be characterized by the loss of all but the most general (most frequently used) words in the language. Goehl (1960) gave thirteen aphasic subjects learning trials on word lists with word frequency and word length as variables. Results showed the aphasic subject's apparent bias to respond in favor of frequently used words. Siegel (1959) found that dysphasic subjects make more speech errors on words occurring infrequently in the language than on those occurring frequently.

Schuell et al. (1961) showed that relative frequency of word usage was an important factor in the ability of aphasic subjects to comprehend spoken words and that gains made during recovery were related to both original performance level and word frequency. Howes (1964) studied 60 aphasic subjects and found that they suffered a reduction in the use of infrequently used words. Bricker et al. (1964) found that spelling is increasingly difficult for aphasic subjects as frequency of word usage decreases. Halpern (1965b) showed that, regardless of modality, aphasic subjects made more verbal errors on infrequent words than on frequent words. Pizzamiglio and Black (1968) investigated the writing of 18 aphasic subjects, and their findings showed that the incorrect prediction of letters is in keeping with the relative frequencies in the English language.

Filby et al. (1963) found no special difficulty with infrequent words in the response of dysphasic subjects. Halpern (1965a) also found that no significant difference existed on dysphasic subjects' verbal perseverations between frequent and infrequent words. A further elaboration of the whole concept of frequency of occurrence is given in the writings of Howes (1964) and Spreen (1968). The frequency of occurrence of words in English language usage can be found in Thorndike and Lorge (1944) and Jones and Wepman (1966).

Parts of speech The aphasic patients' inability to handle certain parts of speech has been noted in the literature on this disorder. A condition known as "amnesic aphasia" has been described by Kussmaul (1877, p. 748), Broadbent (1879), Elder (1897, p. 122), Freud (1891, p. 34), Weisenberg and McBride (1935, p. 299), Nielsen (1946, p. 71), and Goldstein (1948, p. 246). This condition is usually characterized by the patient's inability to evoke nouns. In severe cases of amnesic aphasia, the patient will also have trouble with other parts of speech.

One of Head's (1926, Vol. 1, p. 240) major classifications of aphasia is called the "nominal." He felt that dysphasic patients in this category have a disturbance in the use of words as names and a difficulty in appreciating the nominal significance of words. The patients' vocabulary is fairly extensive and they recognize the objects he cannot name.

Berry and Eisenson (1956, p. 401) speak of nominal aphasia or anomia as the dysphasic patient's difficulty in the evocation of an appropriate word called for by the situation. The difficulty is most likely to be reflected in nouns because they constitute the major portion of a person's vocabulary. These authors state that anomia is probably the most frequent and most consistent of the dysphasic patient's difficulties and usually appears under conditions of fatigue, anxiety, or emotional disturbance.

Spreen (1968) has reviewed the approaches and a number of authors have questioned the notion that aphasic patients will have special difficulty with certain parts of speech. Brown and Schuell (1950), in their early work on a diagnostic test for aphasia, found that aphasic patients had difficulty in finding or selecting any specific words voluntarily regardless of part of speech. Wepman et al. (1956) studied the speech of an anomic aphasic subject and hypothesized that anomia may be characterized by the loss of all but the most general words in the language. Siegel (1959) found that dysphasic subjects make more errors on adjectives than on either verbs or nouns. Halpern's (1965a) findings showed that, regardless of modality, the verbal perseverations of dysphasic subjects showed no significant differences between nouns, verbs, and adjectives. Halpern's (1965b) follow-up study showed that, regardless of modality, verbs and adjectives produced significantly more verbal errors than nouns, while no significant difference was found between verbs and adjectives.

Sefer and Henrikson (1966) administered an oral word association test consisting of 5 each of nouns, adjectives, adverbs, verbs, and prepositions to 50 aphasic and 50 nonaphasic subjects. The researchers found that aphasic subjects show a significantly lower number of homogeneous (same part of speech as the stimulus) responses than nonaphasics and that the word association behavior of aphasic subjects follows the same general pattern of variance by part of speech as that of nonaphasic subjects.

Noll and Hoops (1967) had 25 aphasic subjects orally spell 100 words. The words were 25 nouns, 25 verbs, 25 descriptive modifiers, and 25 nonpropositional morphemes. Results showed no differences between nouns, verbs, or descriptive modifiers while nonpropositional morphemes presented the greatest difficulty. Goodglass et al. (1969) found that fluent aphasic subjects have a higher proportion of nonpicturable and abstract nouns in their conversation than do Broca's aphasia subjects.

A number of studies have approached the word-finding or naming ability of aphasic patients under varied conditions. Spreen et al. (1966) tested 21 patients with amnesic aphasia and without evidence of visual or tactile agnosia. They were required to name a standard set of common objects, and the findings indicated that usually visual and tactile naming were about equally affected with a slight superiority of naming in the visual modality. Goodglass et al. (1966) tested 135 aphasic subjects for their proficiency in naming objects, colors, numbers, letters, and actions and for their auditory comprehension of words in these categories, and in the additional categories of "geometric forms" and "body parts." It was concluded that the pattern of differences in naming and auditory discrimination among words of various semantic categories varies predictably with the major clinical types of aphasia (Wernicke's, Broca's, Amnesic).

Goodglass et al. (1968) tested 27 aphasic, 12 right brain-injured, and 12 normal subjects in tactile naming, auditory naming, olfactory naming, and visual naming. No significant differences were found, and it was concluded that a modality nonspecific process intervenes between stimulus presentation and naming. Barton et al. (1969) studied the word-finding performance of 36 aphasic subjects in three different stimuli contexts and found that open-ended sentences were easiest, with picture naming next, and naming an object from its description last. An analysis of the errors indicated that there is a relationship between the quality of the errors made in naming, and the underlying type of aphasia. Wertz and Porch (1970) studied 15 aphasic subjects in various reading and naming tasks during quiet and during stimulation with a continuous intense noise.

Comparison of results obtained revealed no significant differences in accuracy or quality of response during noise, but reduced latency.

Abstraction level of words Writers in the area of aphasia generally believe that aphasic patients will exhibit different degrees of difficulty in responding to various levels of abstraction. Jackson (Head 1926, p. 35) believed that speech suffered in proportion to the mental complexity of the task the patient is asked to perform. Head (1926, p. 397), an adherent of Jackson, held that the more abstract the things to be named, the greater the difficulty for most aphasic patients. The patient succeeds with the more concrete intellectual task but not with the one that is more abstract.

Goldstein (1948, p. 5) attributed impairment or loss of the abstract attitude in many dysphasic patients to a total personality change, which is brought about by the cerebral insult. Eisenson (1954, p. 9) and Wepman (1951, p. 24) feel that this impairment of the abstract attitude is due not to a total personality change but rather to the dysphasic patient's disinclination to assume the abstract attitude. These authors believe that the concrete behavior of the aphasic patient is amenable to change.

Several studies seem to support the concept that aphasic patients suffer from an impairment of the abstract attitude. Bressler (1955) investigated the ability of 20 aphasic, 20 brain-damaged without aphasia, and 20 normal subjects to solve an abstract problem involving concept formation. The results showed that the normal group had considerably better conceptual ability than the two brain-injured groups. Halpern (1965a, b) analyzed the oral responses of 33 dysphasic subjects to word stimuli counterbalanced according to abstraction level, part of speech, length, and frequency of occurrence, and presented through the visual, auditory, and visual-auditory modalities. Results showed that aphasic subjects made the least errors on words that were designated as a low level of abstraction. Goodglass et al. (1969) found that fluent aphasic subjects have a higher proportion of nonpicturable and abstract nouns in their conversation than do Broca's aphasia subjects, but this difference is confined to nouns in the Thorndike-Lorge frequency range of over 100 occurrences per million.

On the other hand, Meyers (1948) matched 13 aphasic with 13 nonaphasic subjects and found no significant differences in their ability to solve multiple task problems involving various degrees of abstraction. Brown (1955) matched 15 aphasic and 15 normal subjects and administered the Goldstein-Scheerer Test of Abstraction to each subject. He found that no significant difference in abstracting ability existed between the two groups. Siegel (1959) studied the speech behavior of 31 dysphasic subjects and found that they made more errors on words of high and low levels of abstraction than on those of medium level. These results are inconclusive since the variable of the frequency of occurrence of the words used was not controlled.

Goldstein et al. (1968) questioned whether impairment of abstract reasoning in brain-damaged individuals is qualitative or quantitative in nature. 30 brain-damaged and 30 control subjects were tested on 2 concept identification tasks and the conclusion was reached that neither the quantitative nor the qualitative theory is appropriate in all cases since some brain-damaged individuals demonstrate qualitative deficit while others show quantitative deficit.

In view of the fact that the results vary a great deal in the studies related to the hypothesis that the brain-damaged individual suffers from an impairment of the abstract attitude, Spreen (1968) reviews this concept and offers the explanation that other word parameters such as frequency of occurrence should be controlled when testing for abstraction.

Word length During the late 1800s, Kussmaul (1877, pp. 761–765) presented case histories depicting the inabilities of "amnesic aphasic" patients to pronounce polysyllabic words while simple words were not affected. Goldstein (1948, p. 70) suggested that in ordinary motor aphasia the dysphasic patient shows greater difficulty with long words. Granich (1947, p. 11) pointed out that many dysphasic patients are not able to repeat long words after hearing them pronounced.

As seen by later investigations, these earlier clinical assessments apparently proved to be correct. Siegel (1959) concluded that in responding to visual stimuli, dysphasic subjects make more errors on long words than on short words. Filby et al. (1963) compared 10 aphasic with 10 control subjects on their ability to discriminate between visually presented words and found that for the aphasic group response latency was significantly longer for long words than for short. Bricker et al. (1964) administered the Wide Range Achievement Spelling Test to 64 aphasic subjects, and results showed that spelling is increasingly difficult as word-letter length increases. Halpern (1965a,b) found that, regardless of modality, aphasic subjects made more verbal perseverations and verbal errors on long words than on short words.

Wepman (1951, p. 153) and Schuell (1953) feel that at times it is the short words which produce the greatest difficulty. Schuell noted that reading of small words is harder than that of long words because of fewer distinguishing characteristics. However, she has also indicated that a longer stimulus (long word) might be more difficult to reauditorize for the dysphasic patient. In addition, Wepman and Jones (1961) found that in oral responses to visual word stimuli, dysphasic subjects had less difficulty with one-syllable words than with two-syllable words, but they found no significant differences in difficulty when subjects were required to respond to auditory word stimuli.

Grammatical classes In recent years, a number of studies and theoretical papers have come forth that have investigated the grammatical structure of aphasic responses. Jakobson and Halle (1956), Osgood and Miron (1963), Goodglass (1968, pp. 177–209), and Spreen (1968) offer some analyses and reviews of the grammatical concept in aphasic responses. A few studies of this kind are presented here to introduce the reader to this school of thought.

Strauss and McCarus (1958) point out that in correcting the dysphasic patient's language disturbance, the vocabulary and grammatical features should not be taught at random but should be chosen according to a priority based on an analysis of the language in question. Goodglass and Mayer (1958) studied 5 agrammatic aphasic and 5 non-agrammatic aphasic subjects and found that the agrammatic group tended to revert to one of a small number of simple syntactic models, make more errors of omission and substitution of grammatical morphemes, show more steretoyped repetitions of the same errors, make more total errors, have less word-finding difficulty and resemble the classical cortical motor aphasia syndrome.

Goodglass et al. (1967) tested 27 Broca's and 23 fluent (Wernicke's and Amnesic) subjects and concluded that the prosodic characteristics of grammatical function words determine whether they are lost or retained in agrammatic speech. Lecours and Lhermitte (1969), in a theoretical article, point out that the sensitivity of a given phoneme to aphasic transformation is a direct function of the degree of its similarity to other phonemes appearing in the immediate vicinity. Hypothetical considerations of the physiology of language and the physio-pathology of phonemic jargon aphasia are also discussed.

Schuell et al. (1969) studied two aphasic subjects in the framework of generative linguistics. They showed restricted use of vocabulary and sentence types, used fewer optional transformations than controls, and never elected a transformation that added words to the sentence. The frequency of double-based transformations used by aphasic subjects was less than a one-third of that of controls. Syntactically correct sentences produced by aphasic subjects showed reduced semantic specificity. Results are interpreted as showing that aphasic subjects have reduced lexical and semantic options and operate under restrictions of length of unit that can be processed.

From the research reviewed, it appears that the variables of frequency of occurrence in English language usage, of part of speech, of abstraction level of words, and of word length should be properly controlled when studying the language behavior of aphasic subjects. If controlled, the parameters that stand out as influencing aphasic language behavior would be frequency of occurrence and word length.

Specifically, frequently used words caused less difficulty for the aphasic patient than infrequently used ones. This was seen in spelling, free speech, auditory comprehension, writing, and speaking tasks. Aphasic subjects had less difficulty with short words than with long ones, as exhibited in a number of conditions involving spelling, speaking, and visual discrimination.

Difficulty with particular parts of speech does not appear to be a factor that influences the language behavior of the aphasic patient. The naming ability of aphasic subjects has been explored through the various modalities and in different conditions and has been linked to distinct types of aphasia.

The research involved with abstraction level of words appears inconclusive, and further research in this area seems indicated. Finally, the research done with grammar as a parameter is only scratching the surface of an untapped body of information. Certainly, further research into this whole area is warranted.

Phonemic regression Closely allied to the articulation research done in apraxia of speech are the studies that have come from the theoretical position of Jakobson. Jakobson and Halle (1956, p. 74) state "If an aphasic becomes unable to resolve the word into its phonemic constituents, his control over its construction weakens, and perceptible damages in phonemes and their combinations easily follow. The gradual regression of the sound pattern in aphasics regularly reverses the order of children's phonemic acquisition." The statement above implies first, that aphasic (linguistic) can produce phoneme disturbances and second, that these phoneme disturbances follow a certain pattern.

Alajouanine (1956) agrees with the second point. He states that "numerous changes which can be observed during different stages of recovery in our patients are also found in the normal phonetic progress of a child," and later on Alajouanine concludes that there are strong analogies between the pathological phonetic alterations and the first manifestations of infantile language. Critchley (1952), on the other hand, disagrees with the concept that aphasic phonemic disturbances regularly reverse the order of children's phonemic acquisition.

Fry (1959) analyzed the confusions of phonemes obtained from an aphasic patient's reading of word lists. He concluded that his findings tend to contradict the idea that the degeneration of speech in aphasia mirrors (reverses) its development in childhood. Shankweiler and Harris (1966) made a phonetic analysis of the speech of five aphasic patients, and their findings demonstrate major disturbance of speech production at the most molecular level. Maximal difficulty in articulation occurred at the beginning portions of words. Consonant sounds are more often misarticulated than vowels. Fricatives, affricates, and some consonant clusters are the most frequently misarticulated. The most common errors are unrelated substitutions and omissions, and errors were not attributable to specific muscles or muscle groups. Finally, phonetic simplifications typical of young children were observed less frequently than other errors. These findings give little support to the phonemic regression idea. Shankweiler et al. (1968) showed in an electro-myographic study of speech muscle action that the traces showed greater variability than normal in speakers and that consonants at the beginning of words are more poorly articulated by the aphasic subjects than are those consonants at the end of words.

It appears that a number of studies relating to the phonemic abilities of aphasic patients have tackled the concept of "phonemic regression" but have taken for granted that part of Jakobson's statement that says aphasia itself can cause phonemic disturbances. One would assume that dysarthric and/or apraxia of speech components, both of which can cause articulatory disturbances, would have to be ruled out before studying the phonemic ability of aphasic patients. With this in mind, Halpern et al. (1971) investigated the phonemic abilities of 30 aphasic subjects without dysarthria and apraxia of speech, and preliminary data showed that 2 out of

30 subjects showed very minor articulatory disturbance in their free, spontaneous speech, while 28 subjects were free of any articulatory changes.

In this same vein, the whole question of what happens to the speaker's phonology in aphasia and related disorders needs some clarification. Terms such as "motor aphasia" and "Broca's Aphasia" have been used to describe symptoms that may not be aphasia but rather something that we recognize today as an apraxia of speech.

From the research reviewed, it is very difficult to tell whether the investigators used subjects who were not aphasic but were rather apraxic of speech; used subjects who were aphasic but also had components of apraxia of speech and/or dysarthria; or used "pure" aphasic subjects without components of apraxia of speech or dysarthria.

It seems obvious that if we want to discover more about the true nature of aphasia, we must make sure that we are looking at aphasia and not other disorders that may contaminate our results.

Diagnosis of aphasia

Tests for aphasia During the 1800s, the assessment and diagnosis of aphasia was limited strictly to clinical observations. After a while, short qualitative tests were performed to determine the kind and degree of aphasia. For example, the examiner would ask the patient to indicate by fingers how many weeks he spent in the hospital. At the turn of the century, the Proust-Lichtheim Test (Baker, 1954) investigated inner speech by having the patient hold up as many fingers as there were syllables in the word he could not pronounce.

Head (1926, vol. 1), who was a disciple of Hughlings Jackson, devised a systematic evaluation of reading, writing, speaking, and auditory comprehension. He based his test on the patient's symbolic formulation and expression. Both Jackson and Head stressed the psychological components that exist in aphasic patients. Head's test included object naming, color naming, easy reading sections, clock tests, and following directions of a numerical and spatial nature. The sophistication of Head's tests provided the background for many of the procedures used today.

The utilization of mental and educational achievement tests for the evaluation of the aphasic was accomplished by Weisenberg and McBride

(1935). Their test included items that tested all the modalities and non-language items involving formboards, picture completion, drawing, memory, and copying. In addition to the classification system described earlier in this paper, the Weisenberg and McBride study gave us three important advances in testing methodology. First, it was the first study to use a normal control group. Second, they compared performances of aphasic subjects with those of nonaphasic brain damaged subjects. Third, they used standardized measurements for evaluation.

Chesher (1937) created a test to evaluate aphasic patients in which the central features were the common objects: key, pencil, hammer, button, scissors, and comb. Subjects were directed to name objects, read aloud printed names, write names, point, repeat, copy names, and spell names of the common objects.

The Goldstein-Scheerer Tests of Abstract and Concrete Behavior (1941) were introduced at the beginning of World War II, and they were derived from Goldstein's concept that the aphasic patient suffers from an impairment of the abstract attitude. The test consists of the following:

1. Stick Test: The patient has to copy stick figures while looking and then has to reproduce the sticks from memory after looking 5–30 seconds.
2. Cube Test: The patient has to reproduce with blocks a colored design printed on a card.
3. Color Sorting Test: The patient has to sort woolen skeins of varying hues and shades into groups according to different color concepts.
4. Color Form Sorting Test: The patient has to sort triangles, squares, and circles of different colors into color and form groups.
5. Object Sorting Test: The patient has to sort a set of objects into groups according to material, form, and colors.

Shortly after World War II, the Halstead-Wepman Aphasia Screening Test (1949) was devised to provide a rapid evaluation of aphasic language behavior.

In still a different approach, Taylor (1953) describes a scale called The Functional Communication Profile. The Profile attempts to measure the functional dimensions of language performance not accounted for in clinical testing. It consists of a list of 48 types of communication behavior considered common language functions of everyday life. Ratings of each type of behavior are made on an 8-point scale on the basis of informal interaction with the patient in a conversational situation. For example, the speaking section would have the patient saying: greetings, his own name, nouns, verbs, noun-verb combinations, phrases, directions, short complete sentences, and long sentences, and have him speak on the phone.

Eisenson's Examining for Aphasia Manual (1954) gave us a tool that uses the Weisenberg and McBride classification system and evaluates patients along predominantly receptive or predominantly expressive lines. Although the Eisenson Manual is quite subjective in its scoring and interpretation, its portability and screening portions make it a still very widely used and popular tool.

Recently, a number of tests have been devised to put scoring procedures on a more quantitative basis. Instead of correct or incorrect scoring, attempts have been made to scale, categorize, and quantify the different types of aphasic response.

The Language Modalities Test For Aphasia (Wepman and Jones 1961) consists of film strips as the visual stimuli and of the voice of the examiner as the auditory stimuli and includes a 6-point scale for scoring oral and graphic responses. The 6-point scale is as follows: 1.) correct responses; 2.) phonemic errors; 3.) grammatical and syntactical errors; 4.) semantic errors; 5.) jargon errors; 6.) no response, admission of inability to respond, or any automatic phrase.

At the end of the examination patients are placed in one or more of the authors' 5 classification categories of aphasia: syntactic, if the syntax or grammar is disturbed; semantic, if the substantive language is disturbed; pragmatic, if a lack of meaningful speech exists or no context can be found; jargon, if speech is unintelligible; and global, if little or no speech remains. As an added feature to the LMTA, Wepman (1958) suggests an 8 level self-correction and recovery scale as a prognostic indicator of the patient's language ability. The scale ranges from level one, where the patient fails to recognize errors made in any modality and cannot recognize errors when they are pointed out and is therefore unable to correct them, through level eight, where the patient recognizes errors made in both speech and writing and corrects them easily without assistance.

Several studies have developed from the LMTA. Jones and Wepman (1961) performed a factor analysis of 168 aphasic subjects and said that it clearly demonstrated the existence of several dimensions, which underlie test performance of aphasic patients; they argue against the hypothesis that language disturbance after brain damage may be viewed as a unitary, general disorder. Spiegel et al. (1965) classified 50 aphasic subjects into 6 groups on the basis of differences of their spontaneous speech. The findings provide evidence that it is possible, from the performance of aphasic patients on the LMTA, to predict some general features of their spontaneous speech.

The Minnesota Test For Differential Diagnosis of Aphasia developed by Schuell (1965) contains an in depth evaluation of 5 major areas. The Test measures disturbances in the a) auditory area, with 9 subtests, b) visual and reading area, with 9 subtests, c) speech and language area, with 15 subtests, d) visuomotor and writing area, with 10 subtests, and e) numerical relations and arithmetic processes, with 4 subtests. Each subtest contains a number of items that vary in degrees of complexity. A 6-point clinical rating scale, ranging from no impairment to total impairment, is used for evaluating the auditory, speech, reading, and writing areas. Patients are then classified according to the system outlined at the beginning of this paper, and provision is made for retest procedures.

A number of investigations and theoretical positions have led to the development of the MTDDA; they include Brown and Schuell (1950); Schuell (1953); Schuell (1954); Schuell and Jenkins (1959); Schuell et al. (1964, chap. 6). Schuell et al. (1962) performed a factor analysis of 155 aphasic patients on 69 tests comprising 679 items of the MTDDA, and their findings indicate that there is a dimension of general language deficit in aphasia that is not modality specific. The authors feel that there is no support for the hypothesis of a sensory-motor, a receptive-expressive, or an input-output dichotomy in aphasia. A Short Examination For Aphasia by Schuell (1957) is available and consists of those tests from the MTDDA judged to have the highest diagnostic and prognostic value. Schuell (1966) describes a Diagnostic Scale and a Severity Scale to help in the reliability of the Short Test of the MTDDA.

A slightly different approach to the examination of the aphasic patient is The Token Test by DeRenzi and Vignolo (1962), which consists of 20 tokens of varying shapes, sizes, and colors. Patients are asked to arrange the tokens according to instructions varying from simple to more complex, and receptive and possibly other forms of aphasia can be detected. Orgass and Poeck (1966) tested 66 subjects without brain damage, 49 brain-damaged without aphasia, and 26 aphasic patients with the Token Test. They found the discriminating power of the test remarkably high and concluded that it could be suitable for selecting patients regardless of the type of aphasia. Swisher and Sarno (1969) administered the Token Test to English speaking left-brain-damaged aphasics, right-brain-damaged non-aphasics, and non-brain-damaged control patients who were matched across groups for age and educational level. They found that all patients had increasing difficulty as the parts of the test progressed, that the left-brain-damaged aphasic patients made the greatest number of errors on all parts of the test, and that no relationship was demonstrated between age and Token Test scores. Finally, Spellacy and Spreen (1969) constructed a shortened 16-item version with adequate discriminating power and reliability. They suggested that the short version of the Token Test is approximately as useful as the original.

The Sklar Aphasia Scale (Sklar 1966) consists of auditory and visual decoding sections and of oral and graphic encoding sections. Scoring is based on impairment; the higher the impairment, the greater the score. A percentage-of-impairment profile is drawn with no impairment, mild, moderate, severe, and global impairment as categories.

The Porch Index of Communicative Ability (Porch 1967) provides items for examining the auditory, visual, verbal, and graphic modalities, in addition to giving a gestural battery where subjects are required to respond nonverbally to instructions. Patient responses are scored on a 16-point scale which indicates the accuracy, completeness, facility, promptness, and responsiveness of the patient's reaction. The scale ranges from one, indicating no response and no awareness of the item, to sixteen, indicating a complex response with spontaneous, accurate, and fluent elaboration about the test item.

The Neurosensory Center Comprehensive Examination for Aphasia (Spreen and Benton 1969) consists of 20 tests of language performance and 4 control tests of visual and tactile function. The 20 language tests assess understanding and production of language, retention of verbal material, reading and writing. The 4 control tests are designed to detect the presence of visual or tactile deficits that might affect performance on the language items, and they are given to a patient whenever his performance on certain tests (visual or tactile naming, reading) proves to be subnormal. A distinctive feature of this examination is the provision for the construction of a profile of directly comparable percentile scores for any patient, corrected for age and educational level.

In summation, it is evident that the assessment and diagnosis of aphasic patients has progressed from a simple clinical observation procedure to the relatively sophisticated, systematic, quantitative testing methods of today.

Differential diagnosis Quite often the speech pathologist is called upon to aid in the differential diagnosis of the brain-injured patient. His evaluation can help decide whether a patient has aphasia, generalized intellectual impairment, apraxia of speech, confused language, or any combination of these disorders. This information can be very useful, for it helps to determine whether speech therapy is recommended or not and which kind of therapy is applicable. For example, therapy for the aphasic patient involves language training, whereas training for the patient with apraxia of speech might involve a phonetic or motoric approach.

Another advantage is that the proper evaluation of the speech and language of a patient can offer the neurologist another diagnostic sign in determining whether a lesion(s) is of focal or diffuse origin. For example, confused language or generalized intellectual impairment is thought to be consistent with diffuse lesions, whereas aphasia and apraxia of speech are generally associated with focal lesions (Mayo Clinic 1964, pp. 257–258).

Although the literature is somewhat sparse, the difficulties involved in differentiating the four groups have been noted (Mayo Clinic 1964, Chapter XI, pp. 257–258; Darley 1964, pp. 36–40; Stengel 1964, p. 289; and Zangwill 1964, p. 297).

With this in mind, Halpern et al. (1969) investigated the etiology and symptomatology in patients with aphasia, generalized intellectual impairment, apraxia of speech, and confused language.

Preliminary findings of this study indicate that aphasic subjects had the highest overall language impairment but that some areas were more impaired than others. Particular difficulty in auditory retention span, naming, and fluency stand out as differentiating aphasia from the other groups.

The group with generalized intellectual impairment had a mild impairment of all language functions, and this points to the notion that this group suffers from a general "skimming off the top" impairment. It appeared that this group did worst in those language items that were hardest. This would agree with the concept that a general deterioration is taking place, and that the patient shows the worst results with the hardest items.

The group with apraxia of speech showed minimal or no impairment in a number of language items, with a lack of fluency standing out as a differential feature. These overall findings seem to indicate that apraxia of speech is mostly a special kind of speaking disorder and should be differentiated from the other groups.

The confused language group showed a language impairment almost as high as the aphasic subjects, but the confused language group manifested the striking characteristic of irrelevant responses. This meant that the patient gave bizarre responses to various forms of stimuli and showed a disorientation to language as well as to time and place. Since language production and reception involve attending to a situation where time and place aspects are unavoidable, it was not surprising that this group showed a high rate of overall language impairment. The inability to write words to dictation also stood out as a characteristic feature of this group.

Relatively speaking, many a diagnostician has found dysarthric symptoms easily discernible from the language of aphasia, a generalized intellectual impairment, and confusion. Usually the difficulty arises in differentiating dysarthric from apraxic of speech symptoms. To help in differentiating the two syndromes, Johns and Darley (1970) studied 10 apraxic of speech and 10 dysarthric subjects and found that dysarthric subjects erred more by distortion and substitution (generally simplification); whereas the apraxic subjects erred more by substitution and repetition—their substitutions often being unrelated and frequently additive (such as substitution of a consonant cluster for a consonant singleton). They found that dysarthric errors were highly consistent, apraxic of speech errors highly variable.

Audiological evaluation and auditory discrimination in aphasia Several studies have reported on the audiological evaluation and auditory discrimination of aphasic subjects. Winchester and Hartman (1955) tested 10 normals and 10 dysphasic subjects on their ability to discriminate auditorily. Tests of single words were presented to both groups, first without masking noise and then with masking noise. Results showed that there is a breakdown in the auditory differentiating (discrimination) ability in the brain-injured group. The authors state that because of the presence of a lesion in the central nervous system lesion, the figure-ground differentiating ability in auditory perception becomes disturbed with no significant lessening of auditory acuity necessarily present.

Street (1957) investigated the hearing of 90 aphasic patients ranging in age from 19 to 70, including cerebro-vascular accident, traumatic, and tumor cases. 80 of these patients (88%) were found to have hearing losses; 44 of these 80 (55%) had speech frequency losses affecting two or more frequencies in the 125-2000 CPS range and ranging in severity from mild to severe. 36 patients had losses in the high frequencies (3000–12000 CPS). Terr et al. (1958) studied adult aphasic and cerebral palsied subjects and concluded that a low frequency loss of hearing is characteristic of this group.

Miller (1960) performed audiologic evaluations on three groups of patients: right hemiplegia with aphasia, right hemiplegia without aphasia, and left hemiplegia without aphasia. Findings showed that hemiplegia patients with and without aphasia tend to show greater threshold losses for speech than for pure tones. When the patients are tested in a background of noise, there is a drop in discrimination for all groups of patients tested, which may be related to disturbances in figure-ground relationships.

Schuell et al. (1964, p. 186) administered pure-tone audiometry tests to 131 aphasic subjects and found that 87% showed some hearing loss, and 48% showed loss in speech frequencies. However, when the better ear was used as a criterion, 15% of the subjects were judged to have mild, 3% moderate, and 2% severe hearing loss in the speech range.

Hayes et al. (1961) reviewed variables present in electrodermal audiometry using normal and aphasic populations. Because of the problems they encountered in conditioning the aphasic subjects, they questioned the use of the EDR with such a population. Mencher (1967) tested 40 male aphasic subjects to determine if electrodermal audiometry would yield more reliable auditory thresholds than standard pure-tone tests. The data suggests that EDR audiometry can be reliably applied to aphasic males.

Sarno et al. (1969) report the case of a 69-year-old congenitally deaf man who had a stroke resulting in right hemiparesis and aphasia. Investigation of his communication skills revealed deficits analogous to those seen in hearing aphasic patients. Results suggest that the congenitally deaf encode and decode language by the same fundamental processes as those used by persons with normal hearing.

Stoudt (1964) tested the auditory discrimination ability of 13 aphasic and 13 nonaphasic subjects and found that the aphasics did not discriminate as well as the nonaphasic subjects when both groups had equal experience with the task. The author concluded that if "phonemic regression" is found in aphasia, it cannot be based on auditory discrimination deficiency.

Spinnler and Vignolo (1966) tested 51 aphasic, 16 nonaphasic left-brain-damaged, 29 right-brain-damaged patients, and 35 control patients without cerebral lesions on their ability to identify 10 meaningful sounds or noises. Acoustic, semantic, and odd responses were scored, and the findings indicate that the impaired recognition of meaningful sounds (ambulance, siren, etc.) is to a great extent due to the inability to associate the perceived sound with its correct meaning and is not caused by a merely acoustic-discrimination defect. This semantic associative disorder is the common factor underlying the defects in sound recognition and in the auditory comprehension of the aphasic patient.

Ebbin and Edwards (1967) studied 24 aphasic and 24 nonaphasic brain-damaged patients in terms of their ability to discriminate (same vs. different) between 25 syllable pairs separated by two different time intervals. They found that aphasic subjects made significantly more errors than the comparison subjects when the silent period between syllables was short rather than long. In addition, this performance was demonstrated to be related to the subjects' general auditory comprehension ability, but not to auditory recognition or auditory retention.

Although the research findings reviewed are far from conclusive, it appears that aphasic subjects will probably do more poorly in auditory acuity and auditory discrimination tasks than the nonaphasic individual. Further research into this area seems warranted.

Aphasia rehabilitation

Prognosis Before therapy begins, there are a number of prognostic indicators that might give some insight into the rehabilitory process. Eisenson (1949), Wepman (1951), Longerich and Bordeaux (1959), and West and Ansberry (1968) have outlined the following prognostic indicators: 1.) The younger patient, the better the prognosis. 2.) The sooner the patient enters therapy from the time of onset of aphasia, the better the prognosis. 3.) The less extensive the neurological damage, the better the prognosis. 4.) Trauma as a cause of aphasia seems to warrant a better prognosis than the cerebro-vascular accidents. 5.) If the aphasic patient has the will to improve and accept his limitations, the prognosis is better. 6.) If the family of the aphasic patient has the proper attitude and provides encouragement to the patient, the prognosis is better.

Darley (1967) has indicated that the attitude of everyone around the patient should be stimulating and encouraging. In this vein, Stoicheff (1960) investigated the speech behavior of 42 dysphasic subjects following three types of motivating instructions (encouraging, discouraging, and nonevaluative) in terms of number of errors on naming and reading tasks and self-ratings of performance. Results indicated that dysphasic patients subjected to discouraging instructions do significantly less well on language tasks than do those under encouraging instructions. The dysphasic subjects also rated their performances more poorly under discouraging instructions than under encouraging instructions.

As stated earlier in this paper, Wepman (1958) suggests an 8-level scale based on self-correction as a prognostic indicator of the patient's language ability. Following this line of thought, Berman and Peele (1967) describe a method in which many aphasic and apractic patients can be taught: 1.) by helping them to understand that some of their errors are associated with the intended response and that these errors often trigger the response; 2.) by aiding them to recognize which type of associated errors most often trigger the response; 3.) by helping them to realize that they can produce the types of cues that are helpful; 4.) by assisting them to produce purposefully these types of associations and to use them as stimuli for the correct response. In a rather unusual approach, Sies and Hixon (1964) suggest that the word "acronym" be used as part of the terminology in aphasia since it does appear in aphasic speech. The authors feel that the more acronyms the aphasic patient's speech contains, the better his prognosis.

A rather highly organized approach to prognosis for aphasic patients is the one put out by the Speech Pathology Section, Aphasia Research Unit of the Veterans Administration Hospital in Boston (1969). Their work describes a potential for rehabilitation for Broca's Aphasia, Wernicke's Aphasia, and Conduction Aphasia that includes an analysis of the therapeutic set, the auditory comprehension, and the quantity and quality of speech for each patient. From their analysis it appears that patients with Broca's aphasia offer the best potential for rehabilitation whereas patients with Conduction and Wernicke's aphasia show a less favorable potential for rehabilitation.

Psychological factors Earlier in the discussion some psychological aspects were mentioned of the work done by Jackson, who first spoke of the psychological factors in aphasia, and Head, who further advanced this notion. A great deal has been written concerning those aspects, and detailed descriptions of them can be found in the references cited in the therapeutic techniques section of this paper.

One such description of the psychological aspects of aphasia is provided by Goldstein (1948, chap. 1) when he describes catastrophic response as a disorganized reaction to avoid outside stimuli that the patient cannot cope with. Catastrophic responses may take the form of loss of consciousness (very severe form), withdrawal from people, sweating, crying, rigidity, excessive orderliness, euphoria and then depression, screaming, and silence (no attempt at all).

Goldstein further states that the 'difficulty of the task' can produce stress in the aphasic patient. There can be 'psychical' as well as 'physical' fatigue, and perseveration can occur from fatigue which is utilized by the organism to avoid catastrophe. Perseveration is the inappropriate continuance of an activity after the original stimulus is gone. Perseveration can be caused by neurogenic or psychogenic factors.

Wepman (1951) seems to tie up many of these psychological factors when he lists the possible nonlanguage deviations that can accompany aphasia. They are as follows: 1.) loss of attention and concentration; 2.) loss of memory; 3.) reduced association of ideas; 4.) abstract-concrete imbalance; 5.) poor organizing ability; 6.) poor judgment; 7.) perseveration; 8.) constriction of thought and interest; 9.) reduced ability to generalize, categorize, group, or plan future action; 10.) reduced general level of intelligence; 11.) reduced ability to inhibit internal emotional forces that disturb the action of the intellect; 12.) inability to shift; 13.) phychomotor retardation; 14.) feelings of inadequacy; 15.) egocentricity; 16.) increased irritability and fatigueability; 17.) euphoria; 18.) social withdrawal; 19.) reduced ability to adjust to new situations; 20.) catastrophic reactions; 21.) reduced initiative; 22.) disinterest in the environment, both physical and human; 23.) a lack of introspection or self-criticism; 24.) reduced spontaneity; 25.) perplexity (a distrust of one's ability); 26.) automatic verbalization; 27.) impulsive behavior; 28.) impotence (inability to correct oneself); 29.) regressive infantile behavior; 30.) post-traumatic-psychotic behavior showing illusions, hallucinations, delusions, and extravagant behavior; 31.) anxiety and tension; 32.) convulsive seizures; 33.) changing personality profile; 34.) hemiplegia.

Spontaneous recovery Spontaneous recovery is an important factor in the rehabilitation of the aphasic patient. An explanation for this factor has been the concept of diaschisis. Diaschisis (von Monakow 1914) consists of a suspension of activity, which usually arises suddenly and affects a widely radiating central field of function. It has its origin in a local lesion and consists essentially of a lowering or abolition of the power of the central elements (groups of neurons) to respond to stimuli within a definite and physiologically definable zone of excitation. The restoration of function depends on three factors: a) The recovery from pathological processes of grossly organic nature. b) The disappearance of diaschisis and the reappearance of normal activity at synaptic junctions. c) The gradual assumption, at a late stage, of compensatory powers by uninjured portions of the nervous system. Diaschisis can remain for many weeks or months, and sometimes speech never recovers beyond this point.

Recently, Culton (1969) compared the language and intellectual (performance) functions of 11 "recent" aphasics with those of 11 aphasic subjects whose illness was of longer duration. Spontaneous recovery was evident in both functions. Although the severity of the subjects' aphasia lessened spontaneously, the basic form of the language disturbance remained essentially the same throughout the testing period. The first month post-onset appeared to be the most significant period for spontaneous recovery of language functions.

A monograph put out by the New York University Medical Center, Institute of Rehabilitation Medicine (1968) cites a number of studies that state that most aphasic patients experience some degree of spontaneous recovery, which is most dramatic in the first four weeks and usually persists up to 6 months after onset. Sands et al. (1969) reports a follow-up study of 30 stroke patients with aphasia. The authors concluded that significant language improvement occurs after the first year, and patients less than 50 years of age have a better language prognosis than those over 60.

Bilingualism in aphasia Related to prognosis, recovery, and therapy for the aphasic patient is the concept of bilingualism. Osgood and Miron (1963, p. 36) discuss three general hypotheses about loss and recovery of language in bilinguals. These hypotheses are: 1.) Ribot's rule—that the earliest language learned will be the last to be lost (and the easiest to recover); 2.) Pitre's rule—that the language most practiced before injury will be most resistant to loss and recovered most readily (most automatized); 3.) Minkowski's rule—that the language most strongly supported by emotional or affective factors (prestige, language used by spouse, language of childhood, etc.) will be most resistant to loss.

Osgood and Miron (1963, p. 36; pp. 135–137), *Disorders of Language* (1964, pp. 116–120), and *Brain Mechanisms Underlying Speech and Language* (1967, Millikan and Darley, eds., p. 190) cite several studies, such as the work done by Lambert and Fillenbaum, and no clear-cut case can be made for bilingual factors in aphasia. Charlton (1964) reviewed previous hypotheses concerning aphasia in bilingual and polyglot patients and also reviewed a consecutive series of 10 unselected cases. Preferential loss of one language over another is shown to be the exception rather than the rule in such cases, and it was concluded that where such "monoglot" aphasia does occur, it is most likely not due to organic factors alone but to various types of psychological reactions along with the organic impairment of an important faculty.

The value of speech therapy in aphasia A number of studies have been carried out regarding the efficacy of speech therapy in aphasia. These studies are noted in the New York University Medical Center, Institute of Rehabilitation Medicine monograph (1968), and they generally support the hypothesis that speech therapy improves language recovery in aphasia. For the most part, these results were based on clinical ratings rather than objective data, and all patients received some type of therapy; thus a no-treatment control group was lacking. However, two studies (Vignolo 1967; N.Y.U. Medical Center, IRM 1968) did use control groups, and their findings prove to be quite interesting.

Vignolo (1967) studied a group of 69 aphasic subjects where 42 patients received speech therapy and 27 did not. The results for the two groups, based on a scaling of their responses to various tests of language skills, indicated no significant differences between them. However, in the treated group, those subjects who received speech therapy for more than six months showed significantly greater improvement. The author concluded that speech therapy does facilitate language recovery in the aphasic patient provided that it continues at the least for six months.

Sarno et al. (1970) studied severely impaired aphasic patients who had suffered strokes and were assigned to 3 treatment conditions: 16 subjects were in programmed instruction, 7 subjects were in nonprogrammed instruction, and 8 subjects were in the no-treatment control group. Neither programmed instruction nor nonprogrammed instruction significantly enhanced language recovery for the patients participating in the study. Some patients in all groups, including the no-treatment control group, showed some improvement, but this was not significant. The investigators suggest that the consequences of severe expressive-receptive aphasia are not amenable to amelioration with the present methods of speech therapy.

Learning, conditioning, and programmed instruction Recently, one approach to aphasia therapy has been through the use of conditioning and programmed instruction. Several studies dealing with the learning capabilities of aphasic patients have laid the groundwork for some of the work done in this area of instruction. Tikofsky and Reynolds (1962) compared the nonverbal learning behavior of 15 aphasic subjects with that of 20 nonaphasic subjects on a modification of Grant's Wisconsin Card Sorting Task. Results showed that the aphasic patient's learning rate is slower than that of the nonaphasic and that perseverative error was a major determinant of the aphasic patient's lowered rate of learning. In a follow-up study, Tikofsky and Reynolds (1963) found that any significant improvement in sorting tasks by their aphasic subjects was due to the elimination of nonperseverative errors, while the proportion of perseverative responses remained fairly constant.

Carson et al. (1968) investigated the performance of 64 aphasic and 64 normal subjects on 4 experimental tasks. Results indicated that aphasic subjects showed significant regularities in their ability to learn new tasks, to retain their skills over time, and to handle a wide range of complexity in stimulus material. Their slower speed and frequently their lower level of attainment were characteristics that distinguished them from normals. As a group they did not distinguish themselves from normals by inability to perform on any of the difficult experimental tasks.

Brookshire (1968) presented 9 aphasic and 8 nonaphasic hospital patients with a discrimination learning problem in which they had to learn differential motor responses to visual stimuli. Results indicated that aphasic subjects had more difficulty than nonaphasics in both discrimination tasks. Responses of most aphasic patients who did not learn the discrimination were not random but reflected strategies that resulted in substantial numbers of reinforcements. Aphasic subjects tended not to improve upon initial performance within treatment sessions unless either stimuli or the consequences for their responses were changed. In a follow-up study, Brookshire (1969) studied 9 aphasic and 9 nonaphasic patients in a 2 choice probability learning experiment in which they attempted to turn on a set of red "reinforcement" lights by pressing push buttons. Results suggest that behavior-shaping techniques involving changing reinforcement schedules can be used in clinical treatment of aphasic patients.

Edwards (1965) investigated the differential responses of more than 100 aphasic subjects to a "primer" program of automated training and concluded that it was possible to teach severe aphasics any program that can utilize visual discrimination. Rosenberg (1965) assessed the ability of 24 aphasic subjects to make the perceptual discriminations presumed to be basic to reading, after being trained in automated fashion. It was concluded that it is possible to design effective automated training procedures for use with patients who have frequently been considered untrainable. Rosenberg and Edwards (1965) used five aphasic subjects and showed through the use of nonverbal materials, programmed in slow steps, that it was possible to obtain a stop motion view of perceptual skills and cognitive functions such as abstraction and memory. Viewed in this way, aphasic patients are unconfounded by the process of "meaning" in verbal stimuli or the complicating effects of their affective responses when confronted with an area in which their skills are markedly deficient.

Keenan (1966) described a program of auditory and visual stimulation on cards specially constructed for the Language Master. Patients are led by small steps from easy to more difficult discriminations, and finally to speaking and writing the names of selected pictures. Keith and Darley (1967) describe a teaching machine where an electric light comes on for reinforcement after each correct response. The authors propose its use for 1.) visual form agnosia; 2.) visual number agnosia; 3.) visual letter agnosia; 4.) alexia; 5.) visual size agnosia; 6.) visual color agnosia; 7.) body agnosia; 8.) apraxia; 9.) agraphia; 10.) acalculia; 11.) anomia; 12.) paraphasia.

In a study by Sarno et al. (1970), 16 severely impaired aphasic patients were in programmed instruction, and the findings of the study showed that neither programmed instruction nor nonprogrammed instruction significantly enhanced language recovery. The authors describe the step-by-step procedures employed in their programmed instruction for aphasic patients. Holland (1969; 1970), on the other hand, is working with less seriously impaired aphasic patients and is utilizing programmed instruction within a linguistic framework. In her study she hopes, by careful evaluation of pre- and posttest performance, not only to gather data on the program's effectiveness for training kernel sentences, but to find out how much generalization to other transforms occurs as a function of that training. Several case studies utilizing programmed instruction with aphasic subjects are presented (Holland, 1970).

Therapeutic procedures in aphasia therapy A variety of therapeutic techniques gleaned from the literature on aphasia has been reviewed in the report from the N.Y.U. Medical Center, IRM (1968). This Center's delineation of the various forms of aphasia therapy is as follows:

1. Exposing the patient to language stimulation such as watching tele-

vision, reading aloud, and participating as much as possible in speaking situations. Improvement is seen as the result of the combined effects of spontaneous recovery and verbal stimulation, and they are substituted for a formal program of treatment.

2. Interaction between the therapist and the patient with an emphasis on technique rather than content.
3. Permitting the patient to make all speech attempts without inhibition or control from a therapist.
4. Activities that stimulate real life situations acted out by the patient.
5. Role playing, pantomime, impersonation.
6. Conventional remedial reading, writing, and articulatory exercise materials adapted to adult interests.
7. Multi-Sensory approach rather than attempts to isolate modalities.
8. For phonemic impairment, phonetic placement techniques taken from traditional articulation therapy.
9. Imitation practice.
10. Reading words aloud.
11. Speaking practice in a crowded room.
12. Playing commercially available word games.
13. Grammar drills.
14. Selection of a vocabulary based on its potential usefulness in daily life.
15. Use of teaching materials selected according to patients premorbid interests.
16. Conversational practice.
17. Rhythm practice.
18. Training in lip reading to increase patient's understanding.
19. Teasing, playing pranks, telling jokes.
20. Attempts to shift dominance.
21. Singing.
22. A highly structured approach to language therapy based on modern linguistic theory.
23. Building vocabularies around a common theme such as parts of the body or house furnishings.
24. Teaching "associated" words; e.g., when teaching the word shoe, the word shine is also introduced.
25. Using the patient's spontaneous responses as the material for treatment.
26. Singing greetings, questions, and answers.

27. Using a "card index plan" where the patient is trained to write down on separate cards fragments of the theme he has to relate. He is then to arrange the cards in their proper order and speak from them.
28. Teaching phonemes according to the order of acquisition observed in children.
29. Group therapy a) exclusively, b) combined with individual therapy, c) to manipulate treatment conditions, d) as social medium, e) to provide natural milieu, f) for psychotherapeutic gains.
30. Short, frequent sessions rather than occasional and lengthy ones.
31. Daily sessions; they are more fruitful than sessions on alternate days.
32. Full-time intensive schedule, where patients attend language training classes for several hours daily.
33. Language training on a two hour daily basis.
34. Treatment at home to supplement or substitute for formal speech therapy.
35. Patients teaching themselves by following a self-prescribed treatment regime.
36. Use of the patient's intact modalities to teach those skills for which he has the greatest loss.
37. Utilizing incidental learning more than goal directed learning.
38. Direct psychotherapy for concommitant emotional problems.
39. Group psychotherapy to reduce anxiety in order to help verbal functioning.
40. Drug therapy to cut down on anxiety to help the verbal functioning.
41. Reading aloud with and without the binaural introduction of pure tones.
42. Stimulation therapy where the content of therapy is not as important as the manner in which it is conducted.
43. Primary use of auditory stimulation.

Although published reports of therapeutic techniques almost always demonstrate success, it is obvious that some techniques are better than others, depending on the case. For this reason, the choice of therapy should be investigated quite thoroughly before treating any patient. In aphasia rehabilitation, a number of the techniques described can be incorporated into one approach to therapy. For example, this author has employed those techniques listed as 1, 2, 3, 6, 7, 8, 9, 10, 12, 13, 14, 15, 16, 21, 23, 24, 25, 27, 28, 29, 30, 31, 33, 34, 36, and 43 in working with one patient.

A number of pamphlets, texts, and manuals have described generally or quite specifically many of the forms of aphasia therapy as delineated.

These publications include Gardner (1945), Goldstein (1948), Wepman (1951), Berry and Eisenson (1956), Eisenson (Travis, 1957), Longerich (1958), Longerich and Bordeaux (1959), Taylor (1958), Taylor and Marks (1959), Wepman and Morency (1963), Agranowitz and McKeon (1964), Houchin and De Lano (1964), Schuell et al. (1964), Aphasia and The Family (1965), Boone (1965), Longerich (1966), Boone (1967), Vocational Rehabilitation Problems (1967), Buck (1968), and West and Ansberry (1968).

Many of these materials can be used for counselling and guidance purposes with the families of aphasic patients. This area of aphasia therapy is quite important, as a recent study by Malone (1969) has shown. That author interviewed 25 persons representing the families of 20 persons with aphasia. Their expressed attitudes indicated that a counselling program for families should be instituted as soon as possible after the onset of aphasia. Problems such as those resulting from over-solicitousness and social withdrawal can be avoided through early counselling. Problems which have already developed as those associated with guilt feelings or rejection may be reduced, and problems related to changes that cannot be altered, such as role change, may be more easily accepted.

Too often this author has heard—"What can you do for the aphasia patient? Can you really help the aphasic patient in therapy?" It is evident from the material reviewed on aphasia rehabilitation that there is much one can do for the aphasic patient. We know that before therapy begins, there are certain prognostic indicators that might provide insight into the therapy process. They not only provide guidelines for therapy but will also help in guidance and counselling procedures with the family of the patient.

We know that a number of psychological factors may be concommitant to aphasia. The knowledge and understanding of such factors will help in the interraction between patient and therapist. The building and maintaining of "rapport" between patient and therapist is of utmost importance.

Certain facts concerning spontaneous recovery will help to determine goals and limitations in therapy. From the literature we know the best time to institute therapy, when we can expect the greatest amount of language return, and when the patient has reached a plateau.

The work done with bilingual subjects should give insight to anyone treating such aphasic patients. I agree with the findings that show that aphasic language disturbance strikes both languages in the bilingual patient without any preference of one language over the other. Too often, we are misled by the surface pattern of answers given by the aphasic patient in his non-English language. The lack of multi-lingual tests for aphasia and the scarcity of bilingual therapists often forces the therapist to ask simple questions, which in turn elicit simple correct responses. If the patient were tested with the proper materials, it is most likely that his non-English language would be as affected as his English language.

It is obvious from the number of therapeutic techniques presented that a key is being sought to open up the gates for aphasia therapy. But this goes on in all fields of rehabilitation as evidenced by the number of techniques used in psychotherapy or medicine. Without this constant quest for better and finer techniques we would not be on the verge of an exciting approach to therapy, such as programmed instruction, nor would we have come to the conclusion that therapy for the apraxia of speech patient is different from therapy for the aphasia patient.

Back to the question of "Is there value in speech and language therapy for the aphasic patient?" My answer is a definite yes. Although most advocates of therapy for the aphasic patient have based their opinions on clinical ratings and observation rather than objective methods, I would still vote on the side of therapy. I've worked with too many aphasic patients past the spontaneous recovery stage who have made significant gains in speech and language. I remember working with a former lawyer who came for therapy for the first time eleven years after his stroke. A comparison of his pretherapy language and his language during therapy indicated that significant progress was made and maintained. Even if solely supportive therapy is applied and this helps to do away with some of the frustration of being physically and language handicapped, I would say, do it. Why reject any approach that helps the patient on the road to recovery?

On that note, it seems appropriate to conclude this review.

REFERENCES

AGRANOWITZ, A., and MCKEON, M. R. 1964. *Aphasia handbook for adults and children.* Springfield, Ill.: C. C. Thomas.

ALAJOUANINE, T. 1956. Verbal realization in aphasia. *Brain* 79: 1–28.

ALLISON, R. S., and HURWITZ, L. J. 1967. On perseveration in aphasics. *Brain* 90: 429–448.

American Heart Association. 1965. *Aphasia and the family.* New York.

ATEN, J., JOHNS, D., and DARLEY, F. L. 1971. Auditory perception of sequenced words in apraxia of speech. *Journal of Speech and Hearing Research* 14: 131–143.

BAKER, E. E. 1954. An historical development of etiological concepts concerning aphasic speech and their influence upon aphasic speech rehabilitation. Unpublished Ph.D. thesis, New York University.

BARTON, M., MARUSZEWSKI, M. and URREA, D. 1969. Variation of stimulus context and its effects on word-finding ability in aphasics. *Cortex* 5: 351–365.

BAY, E. 1964. Principles of classification and their influence on our concepts of aphasia, in *Disorders of Language,* de Reuck, A. V. S., and O'Connor, M., eds. London: Churchill Ltd.

——— 1966. The classification of disorders of speech. *Cortex* 3: 26–31.

BENSON, D. F. 1967. Fluency in aphasia: correlation with radioactive scan localization. *Cortex* 3: 373–394.

———, and BARTON, M. I. 1970. Disturbances in constructional ability. *Cortex* 6: 19–46.

BENTON, A. L. 1959. *Right left discrimination and finger localization.* New York: Hoeber.

———, and JOYNT, R. J. 1960. Early descriptions of aphasia. *Archives of Neurology* 3: 205–222.

BERMAN, M., and PEELLE, L. M. 1967. Self-generated cues: a method for aiding aphasic and apractic patients. *Journal of Speech and Hearing Disorders* 32: 372–376.

BERRY, M., and EISENSON, J. 1956. *Speech disorders.* New York: Appleton-Century-Crofts.

BLOOM, L. M. 1962. A rationale for group treatment of aphasic patients. *Journal of Speech and Hearing Disorders* 27: 11–16.

BLUMSTEIN, S., and GOODGLASS, H. 1969. *Psycholinguistics and aphasia: a selected bibliography.* Boston Univ. Aphasia Research Unit.

BOONE, D. R. 1965. *An adult has aphasia.* Danville, Ill.: Interstate.

——— 1967. A plan for rehabilitation of aphasic patients. *Archives of Physical Medicine and Rehabilitation* 48: 410–414.

BRAIN, R. 1961. *Speech disorders: aphasia, apraxia and agnosia.* Washington: Butterworths.

BRESSLER, M. 1955. A study of an aspect of concept formation in brain-damaged adults with aphasia. Unpublished Ph.D. thesis, New York University.

BRICKER, A. L., SCHUELL, H. R., and JENKINS, J. J. 1964. Effect of word frequency and word length on aphasic spelling errors. *Journal of Speech and Hearing Research* 7: 183–192.

BROADBENT, W. 1879. A case of peculiar affectation of speech with commentary. *Brain* 1: 495.

BROOKSHIRE, R. 1968. Visual discrimination and response reversal learning by aphasic subjects. *Journal of Speech and Hearing Research* 11: 677–692.

——— 1969. Probability learning by aphasic subjects. *Journal of Speech and Hearing Research* 12: 857–864.

BROWN, I. 1955. Abstract and concrete behavior of dysphasic patients and normal subjects. *Journal of Speech and Hearing Disorders* 20: 35–42.

BROWN, J. R., and SCHUELL, H. R. 1950. A preliminary report of a diagnostic test for aphasia. *Journal of Speech and Hearing Disorders* 15: 21–28.

BUCK, M. 1968. *Dysphasia.* Englewood Cliffs, New Jersey: Prentice-Hall.

CANTER, G. 1969. The influence of primary and secondary verbal apraxia on output disturbances in aphasic syndromes. Presented at the November ASHA Convention, Chicago.

CARSON, D. H., CARSON, F. E., and TIKOFSKY, R. S. 1968. On learning characteristics of the adult aphasic. *Cortex* 4: 92–112.

CHARLTON, M. H. 1964. Aphasia in bilingual and polyglot patients—a neurological and psychological study. *Journal of Speech and Hearing Disorders* 29: 307–311.

CHESHER, E. C. 1937. Aphasia: technique of clinical examinations. *Bulletin of the Neurological Institute of New York* 6: 134–144.

COLE, M. 1968. The anatomical basis of aphasia as seen by Pierre Marie. *Cortex* 4: 172–183.

CRITCHLEY, M. 1952. Articulatory defects in aphasia. *Journal of Laryngology and Otology,* 66: 1–17.

——— 1966. The enigma of Gerstmann's syndrome. *Brain* 89: 183–198.

——— 1967. Aphasiological nomenclature and definitions. *Cortex* 3: 3–25.

——— 1970. *Aphasiology and other aspects of language.* London: Edward Arnold.

CULTON, G. 1969. Spontaneous recovery from aphasia. *Journal of Speech and Hearing Research* 12: 825–832.

DARLEY, F. L. 1964. *Diagnosis and appraisal of communicative disorders.* Englewood Cliffs, New Jersey: Prentice-Hall.

——— 1967. Impairment of communicative ability in patients with cerebrovascular accidents. *Mayo Clinic Proceedings* 42: 648–652.

——— 1969. Nomenclature of expressive speech disturbances resulting from lesions of Broca's area: 108 years of proliferation and confusion. Presented at the Academy of Aphasia, September. Boston.

DARLEY, F. L., Aronson, A. E., and BROWN, J. R. 1969a. Differential diagnostic patterns of dysarthria. *Journal of Speech and Hearing Research* 12: 246–269.

——— 1969b. Clusters of deviant speech dimensions in the dysarthrias. *Journal of Speech and Hearing Research* 12: 462–496.

DERENZI, E., PIEZCURO, A., and VIGNOLO, L. A. 1966. Oral apraxia and aphasia. *Cortex* 2: 50–73.

DERENZI, E., and VIGNOLO, L. A. 1962. The Token test: a sensitive test to detect receptive disturbances in aphasia. *Brain* 85: 665–678.

DEREUCK, A. V. S., and O'CONNOR, M., eds. 1964. *Disorders of language.* Boston: Little, Brown and Co.

EBBIN, J., and EDWARDS, A. 1967. Speech sound discrimination of aphasics when intersound interval is varied. *Journal of Speech and Hearing Research* 10: 120–125.

EDWARDS, A. 1965. Automated training for a "matching-to-sample" task in aphasia. *Journal of Speech and Hearing Research* 8: 39–48.

EISENSON, J. 1949. Prognostic factors related to language rehabilitation in aphasic patients. *Journal of Speech and Hearing Disorders* 14: 262–264.

——— 1954. *Examining for aphasia.* New York: The Psychological Corp.

——— 1957. Correlates of aphasia in adults, in *The handbook of speech pathology,* Travis, L., ed. New York: Appleton-Century-Crofts.

ELDER, W. 1897. *Aphasia and the cerebral speech mechanism.* London: H. K. Lewis.

ETTLINGER, G. 1969. Apraxia considered as a disorder of movements that are language dependent: evidence from cases of brain bi-section. *Cortex* 5: 285–289.

FILBY, Y., EDWARDS, A. E., and SEACAT, G. F. 1963. Word length frequency, and similarity in the discrimination behavior of aphasics. *Journal of Speech and Hearing Research* 6: 255–261.

FREUD, S. 1953. *On aphasia.* New York: International Univ. Press.

FRY, D. 1959. Phonemic substitutions in an aphasic patient. *Language and Speech* 2: 52–61.

GARDNER, W. 1945. *Left-handed writing.* Danville, Ill.: Interstate Printers and Publishers.

GERSTMAN, H. 1964. A case of aphasia. *Journal of Speech and Hearing Disorders* 29: 89–91.

GESCHWIND, N. 1964. The paradoxical position of Kurt Goldstein in the history of aphasia. *Cortex* 1: 214–244.

——— 1967a. The variety of naming errors. *Cortex* 3: 97–112.

——— 1967b. Wernicke's contribution to the study of aphasia. *Cortex* 3: 449–463.

GIANNITRAPANI, D. 1967. Developing concepts of lateralization of cerebral functions. *Cortex* 3: 353–370.

GLONING, I., GLONING, K., HAUB, G., and QUATEMBER, R. 1969. Comparison of verbal behavior in right-handed and nonright-handed patients with anatomically verified lesion of one hemisphere. *Cortex* 5: 43–52.

GOEHL, H. 1960. An investigation of aphasic verbal learning. Unpublished Ph.D. thesis, Univ. of Pittsburgh.

GOLDSTEIN, G., NEURINGER, C., and OLSON, J. 1968. Impairment of abstract reasoning in the brain-damaged: qualitative or quantitative? *Cortex* 4: 372–388.

GOLDSTEIN, K. 1948. *Language and language disturbance.* New York: Grune and Stratton.

———, and SCHEERER, M. 1941. Abstract and concrete behavior tests. *Psychological Monographs* 53: 329.

GOLDSTEIN, L. P. 1964. A case report of an edentulous aphasic laryngectomee. *Journal of Speech and Hearing Disorders* 29: 86–87.

GOODGLASS, H. 1968. Studies in the grammar of aphasics, in *Developments in applied psycholinguistics,* Rosenberg, S., and Koplin, J., eds. New York: Macmillan, pp. 177–209.

———, BARTON, M., and KAPLAN, E. 1968. Sensory modality and object naming in aphasia. *Journal of Speech and Hearing Research* 11: 488–496.

———, FODOR, I., and SCHULHOFF, C. 1967. Prosodic factors in grammar. *Journal of Speech and Hearing Research* 10: 5–20.

———, GLEASON, J., and HYDE, M. 1970. Some dimensions of auditory language comprehension in aphasia. *Journal of Speech and Hearing Research* 13: 595–606.

———, and HUNTER, M. 1970. A linguistic comparison of speech and writing in two types of aphasia. *Journal of Communication Disorders* 3: 28–35.

———, HYDE, M. R., and BLUMSTEIN, S. 1969. Frequency, picture-ability and availability of nouns in aphasia. *Cortex* 5: 104–119.

———, KLEIN, B., CAREY, P., and JAKES, K. 1966. Specific semantic word categories in aphasia. *Cortex* 2: 74–89.

———, and MAYER, J. 1958. Agrammatism in aphasia. *Journal of Speech and Hearing Disorders* 23: 99–111.

———, QUADFASEL, F., and TIMBERLAKE, W. 1964. Phrase length and the type and severity of aphasia. *Cortex* 1: 133–135.

GRANICH, L. 1947. *Aphasia: a guide to retraining.* New York: Grune and Stratton.

HALPERN, H. 1965a. Effect of stimulus variables on verbal perseveration of dysphasic subjects. *Perceptual and Motor Skills* 20: 421–429.

——— 1965b. Effect of stimulus variables on dysphasic verbal errors. *Perceptual and Motor Skills* 21: 291–298.

———, DARLEY, F. L., and BROWN, J. 1969. Differential language and neurological characteristics in cerebral involvement. Paper presented at ASHA meeting, Chicago.

———, DARLEY, F. L., and KEITH, R. 1971. The phonemic behavior of aphasic subjects without dysarthria and apraxia of speech. Paper presented at ASHA meeting, Chicago.

HALSTEAD, W., and WEPMAN, J. M. 1949. The Halstead-Wepman aphasia screening test. *Journal of Speech and Hearing Disorders* 14: 9–15.

HAYES, C., KAVANAGH, J., and IRWIN, J. 1961. The effect of certain variables on the electrodermal responses of normal-hearing adults and aphasic adults. *ASHA* 3: 324.

HEAD, H. 1926. *Aphasia and kindred disorders of speech.* Vol. 1. London: Cambridge Univ. Press.

HECAEN, H., and ANGELERGUES, R. 1964. Localization of symptoms in aphasia, in *Disorders of language,* deReuck, A. V. S., and O'Connor, M., eds. London: Churchill, Ltd.

HOLLAND, A. 1969. Some current trends in aphasia rehabilitation. *ASHA* 11: 3–7.

——— 1970. Case studies in aphasia rehabilitation using programmed instruction. *Journal of Speech and Hearing Disorders* 35: 377–390.

HOUCHIN, T., and DELANO, P. J. 1964. *How to help adults with aphasia.* Washington: Public Affairs Press.

HOWES, D. 1964. Application of the word frequency concept to aphasia, in *Disorders of language,* deReuck, A. V. S., and O'Connor, M., eds. London: Churchill, Ltd.

JAKOBSON, R. 1964. Towards a linguistic typology of aphasia impairments, in *Disorders of language,* deReuck, A. V. S., and O'Connor, M., eds. London: Churchill, Ltd.

———, and HALLE, M. 1956. *Fundamentals of language.* The Hague: Mouton.

———, FANT, C. G. M., and HALLE, M. 1963. *Preliminaries to speech analysis: the distinctive features and their correlates.* Cambridge: The MIT Press.

JENKINS, J. J., and SCHUELL, H. R. 1964. Further work on language deficit in aphasia. *Psychological Review* 71: 87–93.

JOHNS, D., and DARLEY, F. L. 1970. Phonemic variability in apraxia of speech. *Journal of Speech and Hearing Research* 13: 556–583.

JONES, L., and WEPMAN, J. M. 1961. Dimensions of language performance in aphasia. *Journal of Speech and Hearing Research* 4: 220–232.

——— 1966. *A spoken word count.* Chicago: Language Research Associates.

JOYNT, R. J. 1961. Centenary of patient 'Tan': his contribution to the problem of aphasia. *Archives of Internal Medicine* 108: 953–956.

———, and BENTON, A. L. 1964. The memoir of Marc Dax on aphasia. *Neurology* 14: 851–854.

KEENAN, J. S. 1966. A method for eliciting naming behavior from aphasic patients. *Journal of Speech and Hearing Disorders* 31: 261–266.

——— 1968. The nature of receptive and expressive impairments in aphasia. *Journal of Speech and Hearing Research* 33: 20–25.

KEITH, R. L., and DARLEY, F. L. 1967. The use of a specific electric board in rehabilitation of the aphasic patient. *Journal of Speech and Hearing Disorders* 32: 148–153.

KENDRICK, D. C. 1965. Speech and learning in the diagnosis of diffuse brain damage in elderly subjects: a Bayesian statistical approach. *British Journal of the Society of Clinical Psychology* 4: 141–148.

KIMURA, D. 1967. Functional asymmetry of the brain in dichotic listening. *Cortex* 3: 163–178.

KUSSMAUL, A. 1877. Disturbances of speech, in *Cyclopaedia of the Practice of Medicine,* Ziemssen, H. V., ed. New York: Wood and Co.

Lecours, A., and Lhermitte, F. 1969. Phonemic paraphasias: linguistic structures and tentative hypotheses. *Cortex* 5: 193–228.

Lenneberg, E. 1967. *Biological foundations of language.* New York: Wiley and Sons.

Longerich, M. C. 1958. *Manual for the aphasic patient.* New York: The Macmillan Co.

——— 1966. *Longerich aphasia therapy set.* Los Angeles.

———, and Bordeaux, J. 1959. *Aphasia therapeutics.* New York: The Macmillan Co.

Luria, A. R. 1964. Factors and forms of aphasia, in *Disorders of language,* deReuck, A. V. S., and O'Connor, M., eds. London: Churchill, Ltd.

——— 1970. *Traumatic aphasia.* The Hague: Mouton.

Malone, R. 1969. Expressed attitudes of families of aphasics. *Journal of Speech and Hearing Disorders* 34: 146–151.

Mayo Clinic Sections of Neurology and Section of Physiology. 1964. *Clinical examinations in neurology.* Philadelphia: Saunders.

Mencher, G. 1967. The reliability of electrodermal audiometry with aphasic adults. *Journal of Speech and Hearing Research* 10: 328–332.

Meyers, R. 1948. Relation of thinking and language. *Archives of Neurological Psychology* 60: 119–139.

Miller, M. 1960. Audiologic evaluation of aphasic patients. *Journal of Speech and Hearing Disorders* 25: 333–339.

Millikan, C., and Darley, F. L., eds. 1967. *Brain mechanisms underlying speech and language.* New York: Grune and Stratton.

Milner, B., Branch, C., and Rasmussen, T. 1964. Observations on cerebral dominance, in *Disorders of language,* deReuck, A. V. S., and O'Connor, M., eds. London: Churchill, Ltd.

Monakow, C. von. 1914. *Die Lokalisation im Grosshirn.* Wiesbaden: Bergmann.

New York University Medical Center. 1968. *Speech therapy and language recovery in severe aphasia.* Institute of Rehabilitation Medicine.

Nielsen, J. 1946. *Agnosia, apraxia, aphasia.* New York: Hoeber.

Noll, J. D., and Hoops, H. R. 1967. Aphasic grammatical involvement as indicated by spelling ability. *Cortex* 3: 419–432.

OLSEN, C. W. 1963. The dignity of the man. *Bulletin of the Los Angeles Neurological Society* 28: 179–190.

ORGASS, B., and POECK, K. 1966. Clinical validation of a new test for aphasia. *Cortex* 2: 222–243

OSGOOD, C. E., and MIRON, M. S. 1963. *Approaches to the study of aphasia.* Urbana: Univ. of Illinois Press.

PENFIELD, W., and ROBERTS, L. 1959. *Speech and brain mechanisms.* Princeton Univ. Press.

PIZZAMIGLIA, L., and BLACK, J. 1968. Phonic trends in the writing of aphasic patients. *Journal of Speech and Hearing Research* 2: 77–84.

POECK, K., and ORGASS, B. 1966. Gerstmann's syndrome and aphasia. *Cortex* 2: 421–437.

PORCH, B. 1967. *The Porch index of communicative ability.* Palo Alto: Consulting Psychological Press.

QUADFASEL, F. A. 1968. Aspects of the life and work of Kurt Goldstein. *Cortex* 4: 113–124.

RICHARDSON, D., and KNIGHTS, R. 1970. A bibliography on dichotic listening. *Cortex* 6: 236–240.

RIESE, W. 1965. The sources of Hughlings Jackson's view on aphasia. *Brain* 88: 811–822.

RIOCH, D. M., and WEINSTEIN, E. A., eds. 1964. *Disorders of communication.* Baltimore: Williams and Wilkins.

ROLNICK, M., and HOOPS, H. R. 1969. Aphasia as seen by the aphasic. *Journal of Speech and Hearing Disorders* 34: 48–53.

ROSENBERG, B. 1965. The performance of aphasics in automated visuo-perceptual discrimination, training and transfer tasks. *Journal of Speech and Hearing Research* 8: 165–181.

———, and EDWARDS, A. E. 1965. An automated multiple response alternative training program for use with aphasics. *Journal of Speech and Hearing Research* 8: 415–419.

ROSSI, G., and ROSSADINI, G. 1967. Experimental analysis of cerebral dominance in man, in *Brain mechanisms underlying speech and language,* Millikan, C., and DARLEY, F. L., eds. New York: Grune and Stratton.

RUBINO, C. A. 1970. Hemispheric lateralization of visual perception. *Cortex* 4: 102–120.

RUSSEL, W., and ESPIR, M. L. E. 1961. *Traumatic aphasia.* London: Oxford Univ. Press.

SANDS, E., SARNO, M., and SHANKWEILER, D. 1969. Long term assessment of language function in aphasia. *Archives of Physical Medicine and Rehabilitation* 50: 202–206.

SARNO, J., SWISHER, L. P., and SARNO, M. T. 1969. Aphasia in a congenitally deaf man. *Cortex* 5: 398–414.

SARNO, M. T., and SANDS, E. 1967. *A selected bibliography of verbal impairment secondary to brain damage in adults.* Institute of Rehabilitation Medicine, New York City.

SARNO, M. T., SILVERMAN, M., and SANDS, E. 1970. Speech therapy and language recovery in severe aphasia. *Journal of Speech and Hearing Research* 13: 607–623.

SCHUELL, H. R. 1953a. Auditory impairment in aphasia: significance and retraining techniques. *Journal of Speech and Hearing Disorders* 18: 14–23.

——— 1953b. Aphasic difficulties understanding spoken language. *Neurology* 3: 176–184.

——— 1954. Clinical observation on aphasia. *Neurology* 4: 179–189.

——— 1957. A short examination for aphasia. *Neurology* 7: 625–634.

——— 1965. *The Minnesota test for differential diagnosis of aphasia.* Minneapolis: Univ. of Minnesota Press.

——— 1966. A re-evaluation of the short examination for aphasia. *Journal of Speech and Hearing Disorders* 31: 137–147.

———, and JENKINS, J. J. 1959. The nature of language deficit in aphasia. *Psychological Review* 66: 45–67.

———, JENKINS, J. J., and CARROLL, J. B. 1962. A factor analysis of the Minnesota test for differential diagnosis of aphasia. *Journal of Speech and Hearing Research* 5: 349–369.

———, JENKINS, J. J., and JIMENEZ-PABON, E. 1964. *Aphasia in adults.* New York: Hoeber Medical Division, Harper & Row.

———, JENKINS, J. J., and LANDIS, L. 1961. Relationships between auditory comprehension and word frequency in aphasia. *Journal of Speech and Hearing Research* 4: 30–36.

———, SHAW, R., and BREWER, W. 1969. A psycholinguistic approach to study of the language deficit in aphasia. *Journal of Speech and Hearing Research* 12: 794–806.

SEFER, J., and HENRIKSON, E. H. 1966. The relationships between word association and grammatical classes in aphasia. *Journal of Speech and Hearing Research* 9: 529–541.

SERAFETINIDES, E. A. 1966. Speech finding in epilepsy and electro-cortical stimulation: an overview. *Cortex* 2: 463–473.

SHANKWEILER, D., and HARRIS, K. S. 1966. An experimental approach to the problem of articulation in aphasia. *Cortex* 2: 277–292.

SHANKWEILER, D., HARRIS, K. S., and TAYLOR, M. L. 1968. Electromyographic studies of articulation in aphasia. *Archives of Physical Medicine and Rehabilitation.* 49: 1–8.

SIEGEL, G. 1959. Dysphasic speech responses to visual word stimuli. *Journal of Speech and Hearing Research* 2: 152–160.

SIES, L. F., and BUTLER, R. 1963. A personal account of dysphasia. *Journal of Speech and Hearing Disorders* 28: 261–266.

SIES, L. F., and HIXON, T. J. 1964. Acronymic elements in aphasic speech. *Journal of Speech and Hearing Disorders* 29: 186–189.

SKLAR, M. 1963. A relation of psychological and language test scores and autopsy findings in aphasia. *Journal of Speech and Hearing Research* 6: 84–90.

——— 1966. *Sklar aphasia scale: protocol booklet.* Beverly Hills: Western Psychol. Service.

SMITH, A. 1971. Objective indices of severity of chronic aphasia in stroke patients. *Journal of Speech and Hearing Disorders* 36: 167–207.

Speech Pathology Section. 1969. *Potential for rehabilitation.* Aphasia Research Unit, V.A. Hospital, Boston.

SPELLACY, F., and SPREEN, O. 1969. A short form of the token test. *Cortex* 5: 390–397.

SPIEGEL, D. K., JONES, L. V., and WEPMAN, J. M. 1965. Test responses as predictors of free-speech characteristics in aphasic patients. *Journal of Speech and Hearing Research* 8: 349–362.

SPINNLER, H., and VIGNOLO, L. A. 1966. Impaired recognition of meaningful sounds in aphasia. *Cortex* 2: 337–348.

SPREEN, O. 1968. Psycholinguistic aspects of aphasia. *Journal of Speech and hearing Research* 11: 467–480.

———, BENTON, A. L., and VAN ALLEN, M. W. 1966. Dissociation of visual and tactile naming in amnesic aphasia. *Neurology* 16: 807–814.

———, and BENTON, A. L. 1969. *Neurosensory center comprehensive examination for aphasia.* Victoria, Canada: Neuropsychology Laboratory, Univ. of Victoria.

STENGEL, E. 1964. Speech disorders and mental disorders, in *Disorders of language*, deReuck, A. V. S., and O'Connor, M., eds. London: Churchill, Ltd.

STOICHEFF, M. 1960. Motivating instructions and language performance of dysphasic subjects. *Journal of Speech and Hearing Research* 3: 75–85.

STOUDT, R. 1964. A study of consonant discrimination by aphasics. Unpublished Ph.D. dissertation. Univ. of Michigan.

STRAUSS, A., and MCCARUS, E. 1958. A linguist looks at aphasia in children. *Journal of Speech and Hearing Disorders* 18: 54–58.

STREET, B. 1957. Hearing loss in aphasia. *Journal of Speech and Hearing Disorders* 22: 60–67.

SWISHER, L. P., and SARNO, M. T. 1969. Token test scores of three matched patient groups: left-brain-damaged with aphasia; right-brain-damaged without aphasia; non-brain-damaged. *Cortex* 5: 264–273.

TAYLOR, M. 1953. *Functional communication profile.* Department of Physical Medicine and Rehabilitation, New York Univ. Medical Center.

——— 1958. *Understanding aphasia: a guide for families and friends.* New York: Institute of Physical Medicine and Rehabilitation.

———, and MARKS, M. D. 1959. *Aphasia rehabilitation manual and therapy kit.* 2d. ed. New York: Saxon Press.

TERR, M., GOETZINGER, C., and ROUSEY, C. 1958. Studies of hearing acuity in adult aphasic and cerebral palsied subjects. *Archives of Otolaryngology* 67: 447–455.

TEUBER, H. 1967. Lacunae and research approaches to them, in *Brain mechanisms underlying speech and language,* Millikan, C., and Darley, F. L., eds. New York: Grune and Stratton.

THORNDIKE, E. L., and LORGE, I. 1944. *The teacher's word book of 30,000 words.* New York: Teachers College, Columbia University.

THURSTON, J. 1954. An empirical investigation of the loss of spelling disability in aphasics. *Journal of Speech and Hearing Disorders* 19: 344–349.

TIKOFSKY, R. 1966. Language problems in adults, in *Speech pathology,* Rieber, R., and Brubaker, R., eds. Amsterdam: North Holland.

———, and REYNOLDS, G. 1962. Preliminary study: non-verbal learning and aphasia. *Journal of Speech and Hearing Research* 5: 133–143.

———, and REYNOLDS, G. 1963. Further studies of non-verbal learning and aphasia. *Journal of Speech and Hearing Research* 6: 329–337.

VIGNOLO, L. A. 1967. Evolution of aphasia and language rehabilitation: a retrospective exploratory study. *Cortex* 1: 344–367.

Vocational rehabilitation problems of the patient with aphasia. 1967. A workshop sponsored by Western Michigan University, Kalamazoo.

WEINSTEIN, E. A. 1964. Affections of speech with lesions in the non-dominant hemisphere, in *Disorders of communication,* Rioch, D., and Weinstein, E. A., eds. Baltimore: Williams and Wilkins.

———, LYERLY, O. G., and OZER, M. N. 1966. Meaning in jargon aphasia. *Cortex* 2: 165–187.

WEISENBERG, T., and MCBRIDE, K. 1935. *Aphasia.* New York: The Commonwealth Fund.

WEPMAN, J. M. 1951. *Recovery from aphasia.* New York: Ronald Press.

——— 1958. The relationship between self-correction and recovery from aphasia. *Journal of Speech and Hearing Disorders* 23: 302–305.

———, BOCK, R. D., JONES, L. V., and VAN PELT, D. 1956. Psycholinguistic study of aphasia: a revision of the concept of anomia. *Journal of Speech and Hearing Disorders* 21: 468–477.

———, JONES, L. V., BOCK, R. D., and VAN PELT, D. 1960. Studies in aphasia: background and theoretical formulations. *Journal of Speech and Hearing Disorders* 25: 323–332.

———, and JONES, L. V. 1961. *Studies in aphasia: an approach to testing. Manual of administration and scoring for the language modalities test for aphasia.* Chicago: Education Industry Service.

———, and JONES, L. V. 1964. Five aphasias: a commentary on aphasia as a regressive linguistic phenomenon, in *Disorders of communication,* Rioch, D., and Weinstein, E. A., eds. Baltimore: Williams and Wilkins.

———, and MORENCY, A. 1963. Filmstrips as an adjunct to language therapy for aphasia. *Journal of Speech and Hearing Disorders* 28: 191–194.

WERTZ, R., and PORCH, B. 1970. Effects of masking noise on the verbal performance of adult aphasics. *Cortex* 6: 399–409.

WEST, R., and ANSBERRY, M. 1968. *The rehabilitation of speech,* 4th ed. New York: Harper and Row.

WEST, R., and STOCKEL, S. 1965. The effect of meprobamate on recovery from aphasia. *Journal of Speech and Hearing Research* 8: 57–62.

WINCHESTER, R., and HARTMAN, B. 1955. Auditory dedifferentiation in the dysphasic. *Journal of Speech and Hearing Disorders* 20: 178–182.

ZANGWILL, O., 1964. Intelligence in aphasia, in *Disorders of language,* deReuck, A. V. S., and O'Connor, M., eds. London: Churchill, Ltd.

SELECTED READINGS

DARLEY, F. L. 1972. The efficacy of language rehabilitation in aphasia. *Journal of Speech and Hearing Disorders* 37: 3–21.

This article presents an overview of language rehabilitation in aphasia. The methods of controlling the many variables in the evaluation of the efficacy of aphasia therapy are also discussed.

DEREUCK, A. V. S., and O'CONNOR, M., eds. 1964. *Disorders of language.* Boston: Little, Brown and Co.

A comprehensive collection of chapters written by the leading authorities in the area of language impairment. This collection constitutes the proceedings of a conference held on the subject.

MILLIKAN, C., and DARLEY, F. L., eds. 1967. *Brain mechanisms underlying speech and language.* New York: Grune and Stratton.

A comprehensive collection of chapters written by the leading authorities in the area of language and language impairment with an emphasis on the neurological aspects. This collection constitutes the proceedings of a conference held on the subject.

SCHUELL, H., JENKINS, J. J., and JIMENEZ-PABON, E. 1964. *Aphasia in adults.* New York: Hoeber Medical Division, Harper and Row.

A classic text in the field of adult aphasia. This book deals with all aspects of aphasia including several chapters on therapeutic procedures.

SMITH, A. 1971. Objective indices of severity of chronic aphasia in stroke patients. *Journal of Speech and Hearing Disorders 36: 167–208.*

This article reveals the results of a study done with 78 aphasic patients. The detailed analysis of the language impairment of these patients, along with a full historical review, make for a very fine treatment of the subject.